AF243959

When Seconds Count

What to do in a health emergency

First Edition

When Seconds Count

What to do in a health emergency

First Edition

Daniel Hinthorn, MD

Gregg Hinthorn

90MinuteBooks
Atlanta, GA

Library of Congress Cataloging-in-Publication Data

Hinthorn, Daniel
        When Seconds Count / Hinthorn Daniel. — 1st ed.

ISBN 0-9679449-0-2

1. First Aid — Handbooks, manuals, etc.   2. Health General

Contents

What are the signs of flesh-eating infections?
How do these infections start?

Acknowledgments

This book would not have been possible without the encouragement and expert writing and editing skills of many people: Aletha Hinthorn, Sarah Hinthorn, Arla Mitchell, Jeannette Littleton, and Samantha Bottoms spent hours reading, suggesting, correcting and improving the manuscript. Their helpful comments have improved this book immensely.

What will you do in a health emergency?

Health emergencies happen daily, and help may not be readily available. Preparedness is essential for responding to an emergency.

This book provides an understanding of what steps you can take if the unexpected happens. Of course, it is not meant to replace trained medical help.

Empower yourself with knowledge

When Seconds Count is intended to go beyond the traditional first aid books. By incorporating adaptations of real-life examples (names and details modified to provide anonymity), the reader can begin to visualize how they could effectively respond in such a situation. But the goal is more. In each case, we have provided action steps that were used or could have been used to promote healing.

This is not a substitute for prompt medical attention, but a supplement to it by giving the reader initial steps before seeing a health care provider. We discuss when to seek help and what to expect from the health care provider.

In my years of medicine, I have found that too often it is easy to delay action that could have prevented harm. With this book, you'll be prepared to both prevent and react to health emergencies.

What happens after an abdominal injury?

Relatively minor trauma can cause major damage, especially in someone with underlying disease.

A large, high school junior on the football team was a pretty good linebacker, but fever, a sore throat, and fatigue had put him in bed for several days.

A mono test was positive, and he was told not to play contact sports. He understood that he was not to let anything hit the left side of his upper abdomen in the area of his spleen. His spleen was slightly enlarged, and it wouldn't take much of an injury to rupture it. In fact, a vigorous physical examination has been said to rupture a few spleens.

But he felt better a couple of days later and convinced his mother to let him work out with the team, promising to be careful.

Putting all his effort into the scrimmage, he played like his usual self, but he wasn't his usual self. He wasn't sure who hit him, but suddenly he was down with severe left sided abdominal pain and pain at the top of his left shoulder—all signs of a ruptured spleen. He felt dizzy and light-headed as he bled into his abdomen.

An ambulance took him to the emergency department in time. The spleen was removed, and he recovered, but it was close. Some aren't so fortunate.

Dangers from blunt trauma

Blunt abdominal trauma can cause internal organs like the spleen, liver, aorta, and pancreas to rupture. Sharp objects may penetrate any of these or even the bowel.

Older persons, especially cigarette smokers, may have enlarged aortas, the large artery through the abdomen. When these get larger than 5.5 cm, as measured by a sonogram, the chance of rupture even without injury is great.

Seat belts, improperly worn during a collision, are also common causes of blunt abdominal injury.

Unexpected abdominal pain

Spontaneous abdominal pain may occur in several situations including ulcer disease, gallbladder disease, appendicitis, enlarged liver, or in pancreatitis. It is not limited by age as the following story shows.

While on duty in the emergency department, the emergency physician was awakened at 4 a.m. to see a young woman with low blood pressure who was sick, dizzy, and believed her abdomen was rapidly enlarging.

The physical examination showed a tensely swollen abdomen and early signs of shock.

Thinking that she might be having a problem with an early pregnancy, the physician inquired, "Have your breasts gotten larger or more tender?"

"Yes, both," the patient replied.

"Have you had any change in your period?"

"My last one had a lighter flow than normal."

"Could you be pregnant?"

Her response was that she didn't think so.

Suspecting that she might have an early ruptured tubal pregnancy, the physician paged the obstetrician. The obstetrician quickly evaluated and took the patient to the operating room where she found a ruptured tubal pregnancy.

Home remedies for abdominal pain

Usually an operation is not needed for someone who has abdominal pain. Most abdominal pain is due to problems that can be treated, at least temporarily, with medications. For example, for

• Stomach ulcers: try acid blockers like Pepcid which are available without prescription.

• Constipation: increase fluids, eat oatmeal, and take acidophilus with bulgaricus, thermophilus, and bifidum capsules available at health food stores.

• Menstrual cramps: control cramps with ibuprofen or Midrin.

When to seek immediate medical attention

When you see the following signs, don't try home remedies. Immediately seek professional help.

Evidence of internal bleeding (severe pain; marked swelling of the abdomen; cold, clammy skin; low blood pressure; restlessness; thirst; swelling; blood in the vomit, urine, or stool; light-headedness; passing out; or dizziness).

Signs of blood circulation being cut off to the legs (numbness, tingling).

Any penetrating injury such as a knife or bullet wound. These may cause much more damage than is apparent.

Steps to take after an abdominal injury

Most people feel like lying down after an abdominal injury. When the abdomen is injured, other parts are probably hurt also.

If possible, have the person lie on his or her back in a safe place. This is usually the best position if there are other injuries. Sometimes an injured person will assume the fetal position, curled on the side, to relieve the pain.

Cover the person with a blanket or coat to keep him or her warm. Shaking chills do not necessarily mean cold but may result from the injury or the emotional impact. Sustained chills suggest serious internal injury.

Generally don't give anything to eat or drink after an abdominal injury. If the person eats or drinks, vomiting and inhaling the fluid into the lungs can occur. This may result in pneumonia or death.

If vomiting begins, turn the head to the side so the person will not suck the vomit back into the lungs. Of course, never turn the head of anyone who may have a neck or back injury.

If the person is unconscious and vomits, wear gloves or wrap fingers with a shirt to clear the mouth and throat.

If breathing stops, place a towel or shirt over the victim's mouth and immediately begin mouth-to-mouth resuscitation. See the mouth-to-mouth resuscitation section.

Responding to shock

Shock often follows a severe injury, especially if bleeding occurs. Internal bleeding is not necessarily apparent. Shock is indicated by decreased blood pressure; a weak, rapid, irregular pulse; or loss of consciousness. The person may complain of being thirsty.

Make sure the person is warm and comfortable. Loosen any tight clothing, and cover the person with a blanket or sheet. For dizziness, light-headedness, or clamminess, elevate the legs slightly on pillows to help maintain circulation to the heart and brain.

For bleeding abdominal injuries

Control bleeding from a cut by covering the wound with a clean cloth and applying gentle, continuous pressure. Use additional cloths as needed on top, but don't remove the original cloth.

To prevent contact with blood, wear gloves or a plastic bag over the hand.

Emotional Support

Internal injuries can be difficult to monitor, while external injuries can be unpleasant to view. Either way, stay physically close to the injured person.

Keep an active dialogue, but don't exhaust the injured person with chatter.

When caring for a person, calmly ask questions, and discuss pleasant events. Prayer is often comforting at this point. It is important to control your own emotions.

What to watch for

The most common injury to the abdomen after a trauma is a ruptured spleen. Yet this seldom happens unless there is a severe injury or the spleen is enlarged, as with infectious mononucleosis.

Around the house, abdominal injuries may result from being struck in the stomach by a blunt object. For instance, this could happen while playing football, soccer, baseball, or basketball.

A major injury to the abdomen can result from a knife or gunshot wound. The worst problems are injuries to a blood vessel, an internal organ, or the bowels. These injuries can lead to bleeding or infection.

What to expect at the hospital

Initially, the focus is on determining the extent of the injury. Common possibilities include internal bleeding and shock, rupture of an internal organ, torn bowel, or broken bones. There may even be an injury to some part of the body that the victim doesn't yet suspect.

Intravenous fluids, and sometimes blood transfusions, are given at once. The potential for brain injury is checked.

Sometimes the physician will inject fluid into the abdomen and remove it to show an operation is not needed. An operation is often needed for injuries that penetrate or tear vital organs.

What should I do for a rash?

Poison ivy and poison sumac are found in most of the country, while poison oak occurs in the west. After the first contact with these plants, most people don't get a rash for one to two weeks. However, later contact causes a rash in just 12 hours.

A young woman purchased a house in the country. She found a lush growth of grass and vines in the backyard and along the sides of a creek on her property.

After moving in, she spent hours removing the unwanted undergrowth in the yard. However, after two days, she was itching, and areas of exposed skin had small lines of blisters, characteristic of poison ivy.

When a neighbor showed her the poisonous ivy, she began wearing long sleeves, long vinyl gloves, and jeans when working around the underbrush.

Because poison ivy can be easily acquired and difficult to get rid of, prevention is paramount.

The typical red streaks with blisters occur in line streaks as the leaves or stems scrape across the skin. Often victims cannot sleep or work because of intense itching.

Two ways people can get these blisters besides directly touching the plant themselves are from the coat of a cat or dog that runs through a patch or by breathing the smoke of dried, burning plants.

What causes the blisters

The resin from these plants causes a delayed allergic reaction and then the blisters. Blisters are not spread by contact with blister fluid, but result from movement of the body's white blood cells. This distorted function of the white cells may require prednisone (steroid dose pack).

Steps in managing poisonous plant rashes

The first step in managing poisonous plant rashes is to prevent them. To do so requires recognizing these plants. Children should learn to recognize poisonous plants and avoid touching them.

Poison ivy

The glossy leaves of poison ivy grow in clusters of three. The plants can produce yellow-green flowers and greenish-white berries which remain after the leaves fall.

Poison sumac

This has a row of leaflets on both sides of the stem with one leaflet at the end of each stem.

Poison oak

Poison oak resembles poison ivy except its leaves are shaped like oak leaves.

What to do after exposure

After accidentally touching a poisonous plant, immediately wash skin with soap and running water. Also, rinse with rubbing alcohol to remove plant oils.

Benadryl, from the local pharmacy, can reduce itching and allow sleep. Topical calamine lotion can provide relief.

Signs of infection could be drainage, an enlarging area of redness, or fever.

What to expect at the hospital

For lesions lasting more than five to seven days, or for blisters continuing to spread for several days, or if the eyes or genitalia are involved, the physician will probably give oral prednisone (steroid dose pack). This usually gives dramatic relief. Use of topical cortisone ointment does not.

Most people need steroid treatment for at least one week, preferably 12-14 days, to prevent a relapse when the drug is stopped.

Also, watch for signs of infection at the site of the blisters, especially after they rupture. Signs of infection could be drainage, an enlarging area of redness, or fever.

I've taken the wrong pill. What do I do?

When someone takes a medication they are allergic to, usually only rash and itching result. But for some people, death may result from a severe allergic reaction. Obtain emergency medical care, and don't attempt home remedies if someone suffers a severe allergic reaction. Every year, many deaths occur due to such allergies.

One night, a distraught man called the emergency room.

He had gotten up during the night with a headache and swallowed an aspirin from the medicine cabinet.

Suddenly, he panicked. "Did I take the right pill?"

Knowing he was extremely allergic to penicillin, he flipped on the light and discovered he had taken his wife's penicillin.

"I'm having my wife bring me in, and we'll be there in 15 minutes," he said.

He had tried to make himself vomit, but couldn't.

In the 12 minutes it took for them to get to the hospital, his mouth and tongue became so swollen he couldn't talk. His blood pressure was low, an early sign of shock.

After intravenous fluids, adrenaline, and steroids, he recovered.

Fortunately, his quick action after taking the wrong medication saved his life. When they returned home, his wife removed all the penicillin from the house.

Most of the time, if a person takes the wrong pill, it won't be one they are allergic to. It could cause other problems, though, and you should obtain medical attention at once.

Recognizing levels of allergic reactions

Not a true allergy. Most people say they are allergic to medications when a medication doesn't agree with them. They experience nausea, vomiting, or abdominal discomfort after they take pills. Yet these are not signs of allergy but intolerance. Although uncomfortable, this is rarely a health emergency.

Mild allergy. Rash and fever are mild signs of a true allergy.

Moderate allergy. More severe signs are swelling of the body, hands, or face. Even more severe is swelling of the airway, which can cause suffocation.

Severe allergy. The most severe allergic reactions from medications cause the blood pressure to drop so the person goes into shock. Some of the other signs of allergy such as rash or breathing problems can occur also. Unless treated promptly, the person will die.

Steps to take for a severe allergic reaction

Get medical attention immediately because a severe allergy can cause death in minutes.

For the severely allergic person, locate the medicine typically taken for a reaction. This normally includes medications such as epinephrine (adrenaline), prednisone, Benadryl, or other antihistamines.

Signs of severe allergy may begin up to 45 minutes later. These include the following:
- Breathing difficulty, wheezing, or asthma with the throat feeling like it is swelling or closing
    - Dizziness and fear of impending doom
    - Flushed face or sudden onset of red rash
    - Hives or itching with red or itching eyes and sneezing or itching nose
    - Very low blood pressure and unconsciousness

While seeking medical attention, keep the person warm while you watch breathing and pulse. If necessary, do mouth-to-mouth resuscitation or CPR.

If the person passes out or becomes dizzy, elevate the legs 8 to 12 inches if there are no injuries to the neck or back.

What to expect at the hospital

The most important thing is not to wait until all the symptoms of allergy appear before getting treated. The person will usually receive intravenous fluids because of low blood pressure. Epinephrine, also called adrenaline, is given. Other medicines usually given are Benadryl and steroids. If used soon enough, these medicines can be lifesaving.

How do I prevent infection after an animal attack?

Any wild animal that is acting unusual is suspect for rabies. Some animals with rabies will act tame, while others will appear wild. Even in areas where we don't see rabies often, it can pose a problem.

Last year at a home in suburban Colorado, a couple was out for an evening walk. A gray fox trotted toward them from the woods. The fox seemed friendly, and they thought it might be a neighbor's pet. They stopped to watch as it approached.

The wife related, "As it got close, it lunged toward my husband's face. He jumped and shielded himself with his walking stick. The fox didn't make a sound but continued to attack. My husband kept striking at the fox, but the fox bit him on the leg and hand.

"Our shouting brought a neighbor who came with his gun. He was accustomed to dealing with wild animals and shot the fox. The fox tested positive for rabies.

"In retrospect, we should never have considered a wild animal to be safe. Since our dogs and cat are outside most of the time, we protect them by keeping their shots up-to-date."

Protecting yourself after an animal bite

Rabies virus infections are always fatal. However, the virus infection can be prevented with swift action. A home remedy of ordinary soap and water could greatly enhance the chance of surviving.

> A rabid dog ran through a small town biting and scratching everyone in its path. Thirty-nine people were either scratched or bitten before the dog was finally subdued.
>
> Some people did not immediately clean the bites. Others cleaned the wounds by scrubbing vigorously with soap and running water.
>
> Those who cleaned the wounds with soap and running water reduced their risk of rabies by 50 percent.

Several problems besides rabies can result from bites. The crush injury by the jaws can damage the tissues. Needle sharp teeth can penetrate into tendons or joints and infect them. Special antibiotics can protect from the bacteria which infect such bite wounds.

What to expect at the hospital

Rabies shots are given to anyone who is bitten by an animal that could have rabies. These shots must be started immediately after the bite.

Two types of rabies injections are needed: rabies immune globulin and the rabies vaccine. Rabies immune globulin is injected around the bite. Rabies vaccine is given at the first visit and again on days 3, 7, 14, and 28 to provide full immunity to bind the virus on the day the bite occurs or soon afterwards.

Prepare for such injuries by getting a tetanus booster every 10 years. Infants are given the DPT (diphtheria, pertussis or whooping cough, and tetanus), a series of three injections, during their first year and again when they enter school.

How to treat a bite

• Scrub wounds thoroughly with soap and running water for an extended time (20 minutes). Use a clean brush to scrub the area. Don't use a toothbrush that has been used before.

• Rinse well. Don't let concerns about limited water supply reduce the thoroughness of the washing.

• If there is heavy bleeding, cover the wound with a gauze pad or a clean towel, and apply firm, gentle pressure.

• If blood seeps through the dressing, add more padding on top.

• After the bleeding stops, remove the bandage and cleanse again.

• If the wound is severe or the bleeding has been profuse, check for signs of shock.

Preventing animal bites

How can I protect my children from dog bites?

Both children and adults often forget simple rules for avoiding dog bites.

• Do not disturb, try to pet, touch, or push a dog that is sleeping, eating, or caring for puppies.

• Never leave infants or young children alone with any dog—not even with a very good animal, a longtime family pet.

• Be sensitive to clues that a child is fearful or apprehensive about a dog. Even very good dogs sometimes behave erratically when they sense a child's fear.

What should I do if a dog attacks me or my children?

When an animal attacks, it is usually out of fear, sometimes out of aggression, but rarely because of rabies. When approached by an unfamiliar dog, remain motionless. Do not run. Do not turn your back. Do not scream.

If you are knocked down by a dog, lie still, and curl into a ball. Cover your ears and face with your arms. Do not try to kick the dog away. An aggressive dog will only be provoked. Dogs run two to three times faster than humans, so jumping up and running is not a realistic solution.

Are wild animals rabies carriers?

Bats, skunks, foxes, or coyotes are especially likely to carry rabies. Every encounter with these must be evaluated carefully for possible rabies exposure.

Bats are especially risky. When they attach to the ceiling of a room or cave, they may urinate in a fine spray. Such urine inhaled from a rabid bat can lead to human rabies.

How can further injury be prevented?

Up to 10 percent of people with severe head injuries also have neck injuries. Neck and back injuries are commonly caused by knives, bullets, or sudden stops in a moving vehicle.

A 36 year-old construction worker was partying late into the night. For some reason that escaped him later, he and his friends decided to take a swim in Lake Garnett.

Despite his friends' objections, he decided to dive into the lake. The shoreline was several feet above the water which was only three feet deep. He didn't know what hit him at the time. Later, he remembered feeling like he was suffocating.

His friends quickly recognized a problem when he didn't come out of the shallow water. They waded in, lifted his face out of the water, and immediately took him to the hospital.

Their timely action saved him from drowning. However, he was still paralyzed from the chest down.

When an injury occurs in water, keep the victim from drowning. Also, stabilize the neck and back to prevent further damage.

In most cases after a back or neck injury, don't move the person. The neck and back must be kept from moving so that the spinal cord is not compressed which results in paralysis.

Call for emergency medical assistance. Unless you are trained, do not move the victim unless their life is in additional danger, such as drowning. Any movement of the victim's spine could result in permanent paralysis. If help will not become available, strap or tape the victim to a board or door. This must be done without allowing the neck or spine to move during the rescue.

Unless you are trained, do not move the victim unless their life is in additional danger, such as drowning.

Signs of serious injury
- Pain in the neck or back before any movement
- Pain caused by movement
- Possible paralysis of arms or legs
- Severe pain and tenderness at the site of the injury
- Deformed body part

Watching out for the grandparents
The elderly are prone to falls which cause compression fractures of the vertebrae that are already weakened with osteoporosis. They may have chronic pain for years afterwards, but unless there is something unusual about the injury, they usually do not become paralyzed.

What to expect at the hospital
X-rays will be done to see if there are fractures of the skull, back, or neck. Types of injuries looked for are the following:

Torn blood vessels

Chest injuries

Closing of the windpipe by bleeding or tearing

A neurologic exam will be done to see if the person will be paralyzed.

What happens if anthrax threats become real?

During the past two years, terrorists have made more than 150 anthrax terrorism threats. Fortunately, none of these terrorists have used anthrax spores but, rather, used similar looking powders. Such threats must be taken seriously, however.

Accidental release of anthrax spores from a Soviet military facility in 1979 caused 68 deaths. Only 11 people who developed anthrax survived.

Concerns about threats of biological weapons and terrorism have escalated. Only recently have medical and public health communities started to prepare. The FBI now has been assigned the lead role in responding to such threats.

At a shopping mall on Christmas eve in Palm Desert, California, 200 shoppers and employees were exposed to powders. An anonymous caller said it was anthrax. Frightened shoppers were herded into the parking lot, ordered to remove their clothes, and rinsed with a bleach solution. This was to protect them and to prevent them from contaminating others.

The call turned out to be a hoax—one of a dozen threats made to schools, courthouses, and even to a nightclub in Southern California during the winter holiday season.

A Catholic parish in Indianapolis, Indiana, received a letter claiming to contain anthrax bacteria. The letter was opened on a Monday morning when school was in session forcing 480 students and teachers to evacuate.

The Chicago, Illinois, office of an anti-abortion group and a church in suburban Buffalo, New York, received similar letters the same day.

The threats came 10 days after threats at eight abortion clinics in four states.

In Wichita, Kansas, several hundred workers were evacuated, and a four block area of downtown Wichita was cordoned off after a suspicious white powder was found in the State Office Building.

The powder was spilled from an envelope in an elevator. Later, an accompanying note was found describing the powder as anthrax spores. Everyone who rode the elevator was forced to strip, be hosed off, and wrap in towels before being bussed home. Analysis of the powder required 24 hours, so it wasn't until the next day that the powder was known not to be anthrax.

At a school in Lackawanna, New York, two eighth graders admitted phoning in an anthrax threat that closed their senior high school for more than an hour one Tuesday afternoon.

"If they had been adults, they would be subject to prosecution of a federal felony — threatening to use a weapon of mass destruction — which carries a potential of life in prison," said the chief detective.

The release of an anthrax aerosol could allow the spores to drift unnoticed for two to three days in any city. Staying indoors is no protection. The spores penetrate buildings and homes. Anthrax in the air is odorless, invisible, and can be spread by the wind.

Three forms of anthrax

If someone comes into contact with the spores, one of the following three forms of disease would result. Unfortunately, most people could get the lung form, which is the most deadly.

Skin anthrax causes black, coal-colored skin lesions that form if the spores enter the skin. The name anthrax means coal-black.

Intestinal anthrax results from eating food contaminated with anthrax spores. This causes throat or bowel disease. A mouth or throat ulcer leads to large nodes, swelling of the neck, and blood poisoning. Massive swelling of the abdomen occurs when fluid collects in the abdomen.

Lung anthrax from inhaling anthrax is of the highest concern. It occurs as a two-staged illness.

What happens if you inhale anthrax spores

Stage one: Fever, shortness of breath, cough, headache, vomiting, chills, chest, and abdominal pain occur. This lasts from several hours to a couple of days.

Stage two: The victim seems to get better, but sudden high fever, severe sweating, shortness of breath, and dropping blood pressure occur. Very large lymph nodes are found on chest x-rays. Nearly one-half of people develop meningitis. One to three days later they die.

The problems causing death are bleeding and swelling of infected organs, such as lungs and the brain. Eighty percent of people who come in contact with pulmonary anthrax die.

What to expect at the hospital

Seek medical attention within two hours. Starting prescription antibiotics immediately after exposure can prevent anthrax. You cannot wait until disease develops because pulmonary anthrax kills most people after disease occurs.

The antibiotic needs to be taken for 60 days to prevent anthrax from recurring later. Antibiotics used can include Cipro, penicillin, doxycycline, or similar antibiotics.

The major concern is that a terrorist group will manufacture an anthrax spore that is resistant to the best antibiotics, making them ineffective. In theory, this can be done.

Steps to dealing with anthrax exposure

It is now believed that anthrax spores spilled from an envelope causes very little risk. However, alert authorities at once because many police and fire personnel are trained to give emergency advice. Also, you will want legal authorities to apprehend the perpetrator. For your own peace of mind and protection, you will wish to follow these two steps.

1. Shower

Even before medical personnel arrives or you go to the hospital, it is vital to remove clothing and seal it in a plastic trash bag. Shower with soap and water. Bag the washcloth when done. Don't burn the bag because inhaling the smoke could get anthrax spores in the lungs.

2. Seek qualified medical help

Time is critical since anthrax can spread quickly. Since it is a relatively new threat, not all hospitals are properly trained. Ask for an internal medicine doctor specializing in infectious diseases.

Burns

What can I do for a burn?

Once a burn occurs, little can be done except preventing infection while it heals and, in severe cases, skin grafting.

A high school senior was getting into his car to drive home from school with his friends. The day before, he had been on a hunting trip, and his uncle had refilled shotgun shells with gunpowder. Unknown to the students, some of the powder had spilled on the back floor of the car.

As a student in the back seat lit a cigarette, the gunpowder exploded. The car and students were engulfed in flames. Everyone was burned. However, the driver was burned the worst. His friends pulled him out of the car and rolled him on the ground to put out the flames. Their quick response saved him, but he still suffered third degree burns on his arms and back.

Moving the victim into the open is important to avoid breathing hot smoke which causes the throat to swell, suffocating the victim. If lots of hot smoke is inhaled, the victim can begin to leak fluid into the lungs and die.

What to do when caught in a fire

Many deaths are caused not from burning, but from breathing smoke. When caught in a house or hotel fire, breathe through a wet towel held over the nose and mouth. This decreases the chances of hot smoke damaging the throat and lungs. A hot fire will quickly dry the towel so it must be changed often. Because smoke rises, stay as close to the floor as possible.

Protecting yourself from common burns

Bleach Skin may be very sensitive to bleach, which can cause a chemical burn. Use rubber gloves to avoid direct contact with bleach. Heavy, vinyl reusable gloves are often available from hardware stores for such purposes.

Fireplace Sparks from a fireplace can quickly set your house ablaze. Be sure to use a screen in front of your fireplace. Also, a chimney fire may start if it is not kept free of soot. The chimney sweeper is worth his fee for an annual visit.

Electrical Burns from electricity occur when instructions are not followed, wiring is defective, or a makeshift solution has been constructed. If you wish to run your house on a generator, have a certified electrician install it, and make sure fuel supplies are safely stored.

Kitchen Keep hot pans away from the edge of the stove. If children are playing indoors, don't put them at risk of burning themselves.

Hot oil burns are especially severe because oil becomes much hotter than water before it boils, and it does not cool as quickly as water.

> A 60 year-old woman was ill with a sore ear and had been lying on a cot near the kitchen.
>
> A teenage neighbor girl came over to visit. "Honey, would you warm some sweet oil and pour it in my ear?" she asked the girl.
>
> The girl complied. She poured sweet oil into a spoon, turned on the gas stove, heated the oil to boiling, and poured it into the ear as the lady lay on her side.
>
> The woman sustained severe burns of the ear and ear drum and lost hearing in that ear.

How to recognize and treat a burn

Severity of the burn depends on the size and depth of the burn.

First degree burns

What to look for: Minor burns damaging only the outer layer of skin over a small area, such as most sunburns or after brief contact with a hot object.

First degree burns cause redness of the skin without blistering. Only superficial skin is affected. These heal in seven to ten days.

What to do:

• Apply cool water for ten to fifteen minutes using a cold, wet compress. Change several times until the pain subsides.

• If the burned person needs to be covered for warmth, apply a light, clean cloth.

Second degree burns

What to look for: Red skin with blisters and swelling. These take up to eight weeks to heal.

What to do:

• Treat second degree burns using the same methods as first degree burns.

• Intact blisters should not be opened. If blisters do open, the skin should be cleansed with cool water.

• If the burn extends beyond a small area, cleanse with a diluted solution of water and an antibacterial containing chlorhexidine gluconate, such as Hibiclens. Hibiclens is available from your local pharmacy without a prescription.

• Check breathing and heartbeat often, performing CPR if needed.

Third degree burns

What to look for: Burns damaging all layers of the skin making it leathery. The color may be white, black, or brown. Sensation is lost in the center of the burn, but at the edge it is painful. Professional attention is needed.

What to do:

• When a person has third degree burns of the skin, they have had severe airway burns. Inability to breathe may be due to throat swelling from hot smoke. Do CPR if needed, and seek medical assistance.

• Victims of severe smoke inhalation may drool. If they are made to talk or swallow, suffocation could result. Get medical attention at once!

• Soak the burned skin in cool water for at least ten minutes.

• If burns are extensive, the victim will lose lots of fluid quickly. If Gatoraid or other sports drink is available, try giving it if the victim is conscious and can swallow (not drooling).

What to avoid

• Alcohol and injury don't mix. Drinking alcohol lowers the blood pressure and increases the likelihood that a person will go into shock.

• Do not try to remove clothing stuck to the burn.

• Avoid placing butter, grease, or oil on the burn.

Emotional Support

Emotional reaction to a burn may be delayed. The victim's first reaction may be realization of what has happened. Burn victims often have fears for years related to events that surrounded the burning accident.

Your quick and gentle commanding reaction is necessary. The victim may be reluctant to allow examination of the burn and may try to cover the burn with another part of the body.

Five burns that require immediate medical attention

1. Face

Anything more severe than a first degree burn may cause severe scarring. Seek medical attention.

2. Hands or feet

Deep burns potentially produce permanent disability.

3. Eyes

Burns of the eyelids or cornea can lead to blindness. Seek medical attention as quickly as possible.

4. Ears

Deep burns cause deformity and often become infected. The ear drum and hearing may be affected.

5. Circumferential burns

Burns around a structure like an neck, arm, or leg cause major injuries. Blood flow may be restricted due to scars.

Treating a chemical burn

Keep the burned area under a steady flow of cool water to wash away the chemical. Avoid putting anything besides cold water on the burn.

Special burn problems

Burns due to child abuse

Nearly 15 percent of abused children have been intentionally burned by someone. Typically, there is a delay in seeking medical help. Burns that suggest abuse are cigarette burns or burns caused by scalding water on the buttocks.

Carbon monoxide

With smoke inhalation, the potential for carbon monoxide poisoning exists. Carbon monoxide binds to hemoglobin in the blood cells and prevents them from carrying oxygen. So even small amounts of carbon monoxide can contribute to death.

Acrolein

When wood and oil products burn together, such as in a garage fire, acrolein is formed. This is very poisonous. Even a brief exposure causes leakage of fluid into the lungs and death. An early symptom is red eyes that begin to water.

What to expect at the hospital

The burn severity is often not readily obvious. Deep or extensive damage requires hospital treatment.

Fluid losses are common from burns. Intravenous fluids must be started immediately to prevent death. Oxygen and a tetanus booster are given. Treatment for skin infections and pneumonia is common during healing.

The severely burned victim is placed in a large water tank, and the burned skin is cut away. Skin grafts are applied to the bare areas to stop the fluid loss and begin healing.

Why can't I use the gas grill to keep warm?

Incomplete burning of fuel causes carbon monoxide (CO). Carbon monoxide binds red blood cells so they cannot carry oxygen. This starves the brain and causes death or brain damage.

When usual heating methods for the home are not working properly or when you are trying to heat an unusual place like a garage or tent, it is tempting to use stoves or heaters made for other purposes. These are not intended to be used in closed spaces, and they may produce carbon monoxide. This kills people every winter.

After a full day of fishing and hiking in the Appalachian mountains, three boys and their father set up camp in a designated area not far from the ranger's post. After a dinner of grilled fish, they piled into their tent for the night.

Around midnight, the father awakened with a severe headache and nausea.

One of the boys had gotten up and moved the cook stove into the tent for warmth.

When he tried to awaken the boys, the father was horrified to find them unresponsive. When he finally roused them, they were short of breath and moved slowly as they cleared out of the tent.

The camp ranger called an ambulance. The ER doctor said they would have died from carbon monoxide poisoning had they not awakened.

Symptoms of CO poisoning

Early CO poisoning causes symptoms easily mistaken for the flu. However, the symptoms appear rapidly and are more severe:
- Dizziness
- Headache
- Ringing in the ears
- Throbbing in the temples
- Bright red skin and lips

Feelings of sleepiness, weakness, and vomiting are followed by convulsions, unconsciousness, brain damage, or death.

Rescuing a victim of CO poisoning

The subtleness of CO poisoning means most people do not realize they are being poisoned. Even if they realize it, they may not have the energy to get fresh air. If the poisoning occurs while the victim is working rather than sleeping, the effects of the poisoning are more rapid.

The subtleness of CO poisoning means most people do not realize they are being poisoned.

When rescuing someone, be very careful to avoid being overcome by CO yourself. Never attempt the rescue alone. Have someone wait outside so that if you are overcome by the gas, they can lead you out.

If you find the CO victim not breathing, begin mouth-to-mouth resuscitation after getting them to a ventilated area.

Clues to carbon monoxide poisoning

Automobiles

Sitting in a running car in the garage can be deadly. Just because the car is outside doesn't mean it is safe from carbon monoxide poisoning, either. If you sit in an idling, parked car, follow these rules: 1) don't have the car parked in an enclosed area, 2) keep at least two windows on opposite sides opened slightly to allow cross ventilation, and 3) be sure there is a breeze to carry the carbon monoxide away. A running car parked for a prolonged period is never safe if there is no breeze.

Most CO poisonings occur in garages with the door or a window open. However, there is not sufficient air movement to prevent carbon monoxide build up.

Space heaters

Be sure to use kerosene space heaters and gas heaters in well-ventilated rooms only. A well-ventilated area allows the air to circulate to the outside.

It was early November, and the weather had gotten cold. Five high school students had been drinking. They decided to go to a home where the parents were sleeping. To keep from awakening the parents, they sat in the garage.

They got a space heater and turned up the temperature because of the cold. They knew enough not to start the engine of a car inside the closed space because of the risk of carbon monoxide poisoning. But without adequate ventilation, the space heater resulted in carbon monoxide poisoning just the same.

The combination of alcohol and carbon monoxide left them drowsy and eventually unconscious. Later, each recalled having a headache and feeling dizzy and weak, but at the time no one complained of anything.

Fortunately, the girlfriend of one of the young men stopped by the house and immediately reacted. She spotted the heater, turned it off, and opened the garage door, saving their lives.

Gas grill

Never use a gas grill inside a home or garage. If your electric power is off, it may be tempting to roll your grill indoors, but this can be deadly.

Leave gasoline powered generators outside. Don't try running them from a closet or storage space that is connected to the house. Even running them from the garage or basement can cause a build up of deadly CO.

Other CO producers include charcoal grills, coal stoves, fireplaces (with a dirty chimney), kerosene heaters, wood stoves, and gas-powered equipment.

Install a detector

Install a CO detector, and make sure it is near any possible source of carbon monoxide. Make sure your detector meets Underwriters

Laboratories Inc. standards and has a long-term warranty. Test the CO detector often.

What to expect at the hospital

Delay in emergency care causes brain damage. Fortunately, most who arrive at the hospital survive. Oxygen must be started immediately. Sometimes patients need to be placed in a high pressure oxygen chamber for survival.

After-effects include intellectual or personality deterioration, and some people develop Parkinsonism.

How can I prevent a heart attack?

Heart disease is the most common cause of death in this country. Most heart disease can be prevented by making a few simple dietary and life-style changes. Unfortunately, until forced to change, most people continue life as is. Then when a disaster, such as a heart attack, chest pain, or the sudden death of a friend, occurs, they snap out of complacency.

A 55 year-old man was smoking two packs of cigarettes per day, despite years of trying to quit. When he complained of chest pain, he refused his wife's advice to see a physician.

After watching a news report on heart disease, he surprised everybody by making an appointment for a check up. Two days later, the physician found a blocked left main coronary artery.

He was alarmed to learn that without surgery he might soon have a heart attack. That same day, triple bypass surgery was done.

After the operation, he felt much better. He gave up smoking, ate less fat, began exercising, and lost 40 pounds. He began taking three day weekends for relaxation. At his last doctor's visit, he said he felt like a real person and wouldn't go back to the old life for anything.

The 15 year rule

If a man's parents, uncles, or brothers have had heart disease, he should be concerned about his risk. To avoid a heart attack, he must begin to change his behavior at least 15 years earlier than his relatives were when they had heart problems. So if a father was age 50 when he suffered a heart attack, the son must begin a healthy life-style no later than age 35.

Women need to be concerned as early as five years after menopause. If a woman has a hysterectomy and removal of the ovaries, her risk of heart disease is similar to her brother's risk.

Vitamins for heart health

Vitamin E at 400 IU daily, aspirin at 81 mg daily, and folate doses of 400 mcg to 2000 mcg are thought to be beneficial.

Achieving a healthy life-style

A healthy life-style involves maintaining normal weight, not smoking, and exercising 30 minutes at least three times weekly. Medication may be required to control blood pressure and blood sugars. Thyroid abnormalities, should they occur, need correction to help prevent heart disease.

Despite normal weight and regular exercise, some need help with high cholesterol, triglycerides, or HDLs. These must be measured by your physician.

If your HDLs are below 35, you have greater risk of serious heart problems. The following things can help increase HDLs: exercising, using extra virgin olive oil in cooking, drinking eight ounces of grape juice for the bioflavinoids, eating fish instead of red meat, and taking fish oils for the omega-3 content.

Medications that may be helpful include a statin, niacin, and an antibiotic to treat Chlamydia pneumoniae, a germ that may contribute to heart attacks.

Actions steps for chest pain

1. Recognizing chest pain

Pain between the chin and the stomach is considered chest pain. The "pain" is often referred to as tightness, pressure, or squeezing. It is usually not stabbing, burning, or throbbing, but may be. Severe pain often feels crushing and goes down the left arm. Some people just feel excessive fatigue or shortness of breath.

2. Chest pains indicating a heart attack

Most chest pain is caused by something besides the heart. Symptoms of serious chest pain include the following:
- Pain from the chest to the jaw, neck, shoulders, and arms
- Intense, squeezing, or constricting sensation
- Cold sweats and a feeling of doom
- Nausea or vomiting
- Difficulty breathing and blue-colored skin

3. Recurring chest pain

Some people have a pattern of angina or chest pain in the past. For them, if the chest pain is more severe, in a different place, or is occurring more frequently, immediate medical attention is necessary.

Life saving steps for a heart attack

Acute heart attacks cause sudden death in many victims. Immediate action can be lifesaving for anyone who has the above symptoms.

1. Call 911, and do CPR if necessary.

2. Give one aspirin. This helps prevent or dissolve blood clots in the coronary arteries. In rare cases, if a person is having a hemorrhagic stroke, aspirin worsens bleeding and can lead to death.

Often overlooked causes of heart attacks

Shoveling snow

Often, when a person is participating in vigorous activity, such as cutting wood or shoveling snow, he is reluctant to quit before the job is done. If there is shortness of breath, coughing, or wheezing, he should stop and rest.

Every winter after a fresh snowfall, men with unrecognized heart disease shovel snow. The average weight of one shovel of snow is

15 to 25 pounds. This action repeated several hundred times in rapid succession places stress on the heart. A person unaccustomed to this work can quickly overexert, causing a heart attack.

Walking in the cold

Breathing cold air while exerting oneself, whether walking, shoveling snow, or carrying wood for the fireplace, is more taxing than similar work during warmer temperatures. When temperatures are colder, reduce exertion to what you can do easily.

Emotional outbursts

For many people, the triggering event for a heart attack is not vigorous exercise but an emotional outburst.

A physician 200 years ago, William Heberden, speaking of his own chest pain said, "The person who makes me angry will kill me." His statement was prophetic. During a question and answer session years later, a disagreement ensued. The physician became angry, developed chest pain, and dropped dead.

What to expect at the hospital

A few years ago, the focus was only pain relief. Now, emergency physicians can limit the damage done during the first three hours.

A heart catheterization and a clot buster can restore blood flow to the heart. This usually prevents permanent heart damage.

Electrocardiograms, intensive care unit monitoring, oxygen, and intravenous fluids are started. Blood tests are done to measure heart muscle deterioration.

Our baby is coming! What do I do?

Childbirth can be overwhelming if medical assistance is unavailable. Sometimes even the most well-planned pregnancy ends in an unexpected delivery.

A non-physician friend told his story.

It was 2 a.m. when the call came from our neighbor. "My wife is having the baby," said her husband.

I jumped out of bed, slipped on my jeans, and headed over.

When I arrived, she was lying on a small mattress. Her breathing and sweating showed she was about to deliver.

Her husband was speaking to the hospital delivery room nurse. Turning to me, he asked, "Can you help as I tell you what the nurse says?"

"Absolutely," I said as I washed my hands, pulled on rubber gloves, and knelt beside his wife.

With the ambulance on its way, the contractions increased. Suddenly, with a strong push, the baby's head emerged. I supported the tiny head in my hands as the mother continued to push the rest of the baby girl out.

We still had to tie off the umbilical cord. I removed the laces from a shoe and used this to tie off the umbilical cord. With a dry towel, I wiped the baby's face.

As the afterbirth came, paramedics arrived. They pronounced our work a success.

Preparing for delivery

Before the birth draws near, have these items available if the delivery could occur in the home.

• Suction bulb for clearing mucus and blood from the baby's nose and mouth
  • Sterile rubber gloves to wear while assisting the delivery
  • Blankets for mother and baby
  • Diaper
  • Sterile scissors
  • Two clean cords to tie the umbilical cord

Delivering the baby

If the baby will be delivered at home instead of in the hospital, the following steps will be important.

1. Care for the mother

Provide for the mother's emotional well-being. Encourage her to breathe deeply and slowly, especially during contractions.

2. Support the baby's head

Support the head after it comes through the birth canal while asking the mother to push. The baby will naturally turn to one side. Use a towel to hold the baby because the baby will be slippery.

3. Clear the airway

Use the suction bulb to clean out the baby's nose and mouth as soon as possible. If no suction bulb is available, use a dry towel to clean the mouth.

If the umbilical cord is around the neck, gently slip it over the baby's head. Do not pull on the cord.

4. Let fluids drain

Once delivered, use a towel to hold the baby's face down with the feet above the head for a few seconds.

Allow the fluids to drain. Use the suction bulb to remove fluids again from the nose and mouth. This stimulates breathing.

5. Check breathing

If the baby is not breathing, flick the soles of its feet. Rarely is mouth-to-mouth resuscitation needed.

After it starts crying, dry the baby. Place it face down on the mother's chest to allow the baby to nurse. This helps to expel the placenta.

6. Tie the umbilical cord

If medical help is not available, you will need to tie the umbilical cord after the baby is completely out of the birth canal.

• Use a clean, strong string to tie around the cord no closer than four inches to the baby. If a shoelace will be used, boil it for 20 minutes for sterility.

• Tie a second string around the umbilical cord four inches from the first knot, eight inches from the baby.

• Use strong knots in both places. A loose knot can allow the baby to bleed to death after the cord is cut.

• Using sterile scissors or a heated knife blade, cut the cord between the two knots. It should only bleed for a few seconds.

• Wrap the end of the cord attached to the baby in sterile gauze or a clean dry cloth.

Expect contractions to continue until the placenta is delivered.

5. Care for the mother after the birth

Expect contractions to continue until the placenta is delivered. Put it in a plastic bag. Help her clean with soap and water.

Emotional support

During labor

The mother's help is mandatory throughout the delivery. Communicate with her in a calm, supportive voice. Encourage her to breathe deeply and slowly during contractions. Allow her to squeeze someone's hand during a contraction.

After delivery

The overwhelming fatigue that follows a birth may cause the mother to fall asleep immediately. If she is awake and breast feeding, keep her comfortable.

What not to do during childbirth

Do not try to stop the birth.

Do not let anyone with an infection, skin lesions, a cough, or other illness near the mother or baby.

Do not pull the baby from the birth canal.

Do not pull on the umbilical cord.

Do not permit the mother to go to the bathroom during the last stages of labor.

Help! His heart is not beating.

Of all the emergency techniques described in this book, this one is the most important. If the technique discussed here is not used, certain victims will die quickly. A person can live for 30 days without food, for three days without water, for three minutes without oxygen, but only for 30 seconds without a heartbeat.

During a flight from Atlanta to Kansas City, a passenger called the flight attendant to check on his golfing partner sitting in the seat next to him. The man was in his early fifties and appeared to be unconscious.

The flight attendant urgently called, "Is there a physician on board?"

Seeing a man in trouble who appeared blue, I moved forward and found he wasn't breathing. He had no pulse in his neck and did not respond when his name was called. Opening his mouth, I made sure there was no food lodged in the back of his throat.

Placing the man on his back in the aisle, we began CPR. To begin chest compressions, I placed the heel of my palm midway down his breast bone.

After locking the fingers of both hands so that one palm pushed down on the other, I began chest compressions. The distance I pressed down was a little more than the width of a golf ball. I made sure I kept my hands in contact with his chest between compressions.

I paused after every 15 chest compressions long enough to clamp his nose and give two full breaths into his mouth.

This sequence of breathing and compressing his chest continued for 20 minutes. Fortunately, he was alive when the plane landed and a Life Flight helicopter took him to a nearby hospital.

Defibrillator

Prompt use of a defibrillator gives the best chance for survival after the heart stops. On this airplane, a defibrillator was not available. However, on many planes they are.

While getting the defibrillator

Begin CPR to prevent acid build up from lack of oxygen. This will help the victim respond when the electric shock is given.

Defibrillators for general use are fairly foolproof so that if the electrodes are placed on a person whose heart is beating, no electrical discharge will occur.

If the victim lacks breathing and heartbeat, restarting the heartbeat at once dramatically increases the chances of the person living. For every minute of delay before the person is shocked, the chance of survival drops by ten percent.

Be sure no one touches the victim when the electric shock is given or their heart may stop beating.

Save a life with CPR

When a person appears unconscious, has no pulse in the neck, and does not appear to be breathing, tell the nearest person to call 911 while you begin CPR.

Do the ABCs before CPR

Airway. Open the mouth and be sure no food is blocking the airway. (If there could be a neck injury, don't do this.)

Breathing. Look for breathing. Place your ear close to the nose and mouth to listen and feel for breathing.

Circulation. Use two fingers to check for a pulse between the Adam's apple and the muscle on the side of the neck.

The CPR rule of thumb: 15 and 2, when they're blue
(15 chest compressions followed by 2 full breaths)

1. If the victim has a pulse but is not breathing, begin mouth-to-mouth resuscitation without chest compressions after being sure there is nothing caught in the throat.

With the victim on his back on a firm surface, shout his name, recheck the pulse and respirations. If this does not rouse the person, lightly tap him.

Lift the chin while tilting the head back. (Don't do this if there could be a neck injury.)

> Be careful. An intern did this to a patient after a nurse called a CODE BLUE. The intern did not check for pulse before starting CPR. The "dead man" immediately slugged him in the jaw.

2. Lift the chin while tilting the head back. (Don't do this if there could be a neck injury.)

3. If there are no respirations, pinch the victim's nostrils together. Take a deep breath and seal your lips over the victim's mouth. Blow two breaths. After each breath, release the seal of your lips from the victim's mouth to allow him to exhale.

If the chest does not rise with each breath, extend the head back further. The airway may be blocked, or you may be blowing air into the stomach instead of the lungs. If the stomach becomes filled with air, the person may vomit, causing suffocation. If vomiting occurs, turn the victim on his side so the vomit will exit the mouth.

4. Kneeling at the person's right side, locate the notch at the lower end of the breast bone. Two finger widths above the notch, place the heel of your left palm on the breast bone. *Note: Stop here if the victim is under age 8 or under 80 pounds. See the steps for child CPR.*

5. Lean over the victim's chest, and place the heel of your right hand on top of the other hand. Sharply push the breast bone down 1 to 1.5 inches and let up.

6. Continue to lean over the person with your shoulders directly above their body. Keep your arms straight and locked.

7. Use straight down pressure with both arms to push the breast bone against the heart. Compress 15 times. Count out loud, saying, "One-and-two-and-three-and..." up to 15. Push on the numbers and release on the "and."

8. At 15, stop the compressions, and give two full breaths into the victim's mouth.

9. Repeat this 15-to-2 cycle until help arrives or the victim has a pulse and is breathing.

10. Each minute, do 80 to 100 compressions. Check for pulse after each minute of compressions.

CPR for children ages 1 to 8

1. Use only one hand to compress. Place the other hand on the forehead to tilt the head back to open the airway while you are compressing the chest. (Again, don't tilt the head back if the victim has a neck injury.)

2. Keep your fingers off the child's chest. Use only the heel of the palm with straight down pressure.

3. Compress the breast bone one inch. People who are not familiar with CPR push too hard.

4. Perform chest compressions 80 times per minute.

5. After five compressions, give two slow breaths into the child's mouth. Repeat the cycle. After each minute, check for a pulse.

6. Continue until the child has a heartbeat and is breathing or until help arrives.

TIP: If there are two rescuers

• If the first rescuer is tired, have the second rescuer take over when the first rescuer is ready to give the breaths.

• Have one rescuer check to be sure compressions and respirations are adequate by watching the chest rise and fall and feeling the neck artery.

• If the second rescuer detects a pulse during each chest compression but not when you stop, this is a sign of good CPR. Continue CPR. If there is a pulse without compressions, see if breathing also occurs. If so, stop CPR.

CPR for an infant

Feel carefully for a heartbeat near the left nipple. If there is a heartbeat but no breathing, use mouth-to-mouth resuscitation. If there is no heartbeat, begin CPR immediately.

If the infant is not breathing

Lay the infant face up. Shake or tap hard on the bottom of the foot to rouse the infant. Clear the airway, and remove any foreign objects from the mouth.

Lift the chin to extend the neck while supporting both. Do not tilt the head at all if you suspect neck injuries.

1. Seal your mouth over both the infant's mouth and nose.

2. Blow two small puffs of air very slowly, using only the air in your mouth.

3. Try to find a pulse on the inside of the elbow or on the side of the neck below the jaw.

4. If the infant has a pulse but breathing is weak or absent, continue only mouth-to-mouth resuscitation at 20 breaths per minute until the infant revives.

If the infant does not have a pulse

1. Spread one hand over the infant's chest so that your thumb is at the base of the throat and your little finger is at the end of the breastbone.

2. Keep your index finger and middle finger together and lift the others from the chest.

3. Use the tips of your index and middle fingers to press gently on the center of the breastbone, depressing 1/2 to 3/4 inches. Use only your fingers for the compressions so you don't crush the infant's chest. Do five compressions in three seconds. Then do one breath.

4. Keep the infant's head tilted with your other hand to allow for breathing.

5. Perform chest compressions 80-100 times per minute.

6. After every fifth compression, blow one small puff of air into the infant's nose and mouth.

When the infant revives

Keep the child warm and check for continued pulse and breathing. Attend to any injuries or illnesses.

What makes the heart stop beating

- Electrocution from a damaged power line
- Lightening strikes
- Auto accident
- A blow to the chest as from a baseball

• Certain diseases and some medications
• Most often hearts stop without a known reason. This is called sudden death.

Is it worthwhile to perform lifesaving measures again and again?

A 62 year-old man's heart stopped beating several times each day while in the hospital ICU. Each time, defibrillator paddles were applied, restarting his heart.

After 85 such episodes of "dying" the man's heart returned to a normal beat. He walked out of the hospital in good shape.

On another note, restarting the heart with a defibrillator is painful. Each time the cardiac monitor alarm sounded, electrical defibrillator paddles were applied to his chest, shocking him back to a normal heartbeat.

On one occasion, the shock was given before he lost consciousness, causing extreme pain. After that, he raised his hands holding off the paddles until losing consciousness, saving himself from feeling the jolt.

CAUTION: Because CPR is complicated, every family should have at least two members take a CPR class. The life of someone you love might be saved because of this investment of time. Once you have the training, share it with others.

How should I do mouth-to-mouth breathing if someone may be carrying a disease?

A physician called me recently. He had been called to the hospital room of a person found lying on the floor without pulse and not breathing.

He wisely placed a thin towel over the person's face before he began to do mouth-to-mouth breathing. He successfully restored the person back to normal breathing and heartbeat.

Review of the patient's record showed the man had AIDS.

The physician asked, "Was I exposed to HIV, and should I take medications?"

Since there was no bleeding, and since the towel had absorbed all the secretions, we decided he had not been exposed to the HIV virus.

The use of a towel or other cloth material, such as a cloth napkin, tablecloth, cotton shirt, or sweater, will greatly reduce the possibility of disease transmission during mouth-to-mouth breathing.

What should I do if my child is choking?

A mother recently related how she had to react instantly to save the life of her child.

Her family was just sitting down at the dinner table when she noticed something unusual about her daughter.

The sister had cut up a canned peach for the three year-old. She had been happily eating and talking. But as they sat down, she was strangely silent.

The mother quickly moved around the table to the high chair, sensing something was wrong. The little girl's eyes pleaded, yet she said nothing.

The mother placed her arms around her to do the Heimlich Maneuver. She gave a gentle squeeze. Nothing happened. Again she squeezed—this time a little more sharply.

A peach slice shot out of her mouth across the table.

As she gave her a long hug, the reality of what almost happened left her shaking. No ambulance would have ever arrived in time to save her beautiful, little girl. Only the mother could have responded.

What to do when a child is choking

The mother reacted quickly and most likely saved her child's life. If there is time, however, first do the following steps for a child under 100 pounds. It is better to avoid the Heimlich maneuver, if possible, since it can break a child's ribs. Of course, it's better to have broken ribs than to lose a life.

The steps before doing a Heimlich maneuver are the following:

• Hold the child's head down over your arm.

• Keep the child's head lower than their body.

• Administer a sharp blow between their shoulder blades with the palm of your hand. If not successful, repeat this step.

Performing the Heimlich maneuver on children or adults

1. From behind, wrap your arms around the victim.
2. Make a fist with one hand, and cover it with the other hand.
3. Place the top of your fist just above the person's navel but below their rib cage.

Note: for pregnant women or very large people, place the arms around the middle of the chest.

4. Thrust fists back and up.
5. Repeat several times, if necessary.

If the person has a neck injury, don't move the victim since it could cause paralysis if the spinal cord is compressed.

What to do if alone when choking

The inability to breathe is terrifying. Here's what you should do if you are alone and begin to choke.

First, dial 911 even if you are unable to speak.

Second, do the Heimlich maneuver on yourself. Bend over the back of a tall chair or counter top, and press forcefully at the level of your belly button.

Third, if the Heimlich maneuver fails, place a finger in the back of the throat to hook the food and dislodge it.

It is better to avoid the Heimlich maneuver, if possible, since it can break a child's ribs. Of course, it's better to have broken ribs than to lose a life.

One person choking while alone folded his fists and thrust them into the pit of his stomach. That didn't work, so he allowed himself to fall face down over the back of a chair. It required three attempts, but ultimately the food flew out. Had it not, he could have formed his index finger into a J shape and attempted to dislodge the food.

Signs of something caught in the throat

The victim may not make gagging noises. While these noises sometimes occur, some victims, particularly children, simply cease speaking and turn blue or ash-colored, called cyanosis. Look for any one of the following four signs:
- Clutching the throat
- Cough which leads to a gasp and an inability to speak
- Sudden loss of consciousness while eating
- Gray or blue lips, fingernails, skin, and gums

Emergency Choking Tip: Never give the choking person a piece of soft bread to help dislodge the food. This could cause the trapped food to fall further back into the throat.

Why am I waking up short of breath?

Congestive heart failure is one of the most common reasons for hospitalization. Congestive heart failure occurs when the heart no longer pumps the blood needed by the body.

A 65 year-old diabetic came into the emergency room at 4 a.m. He complained of awakening during the night feeling short of breath. He had sat up to breathe and said he felt very wheezy, like he might be going to die. He said it felt better when he opened the window. He had also recently experienced breathlessness when he climbed even a few steps. The cold, blowing air awakened his wife who insisted he go to the hospital.

Congestive heart failure causes fatigue, breathlessness, awakening from sleep, and death. Swelling of the legs, fluid gain, and abdominal pain from a swollen liver are part of the symptoms. If the proper medications are not selected, death occurs in a few months.

The underlying causes are many and include heart attacks, high blood pressure, heart valve disease, and lung disease.

Many people with congestive heart failure learn that they need to sit up to breathe, and so they sleep with their head on several pillows, or they sleep sitting up. They also select a diet low in sodium to keep from having too much swelling.

What to expect at the hospital

A search for the underlying cause of congestive heart failure will begin. An electrocardiogram will be taken to be certain that a painless heart attack was not the cause. A chest x-ray will evaluate for fluid on the lungs or an enlarged heart.

Immediate care includes bed rest, oxygen, morphine for the severe anxiety, restriction of salt and water, and a water pill to remove some of the excess liquid. Other medications needed are ACE inhibitors and digitalis.

How do I rescue someone who is drowning?

Children under age five have the greatest risk of drowning, and most drownings happen in swimming pools. If you have a pool in your area, make sure everyone in your family knows how to swim. A backyard pool should have a fence, child latches, and alarms. Also, anyone who owns a pool should know CPR.

It was mid-afternoon in Westchester county when a mother noticed her three year-old daughter was missing. She searched the house but could not locate her. Running outside, she saw her daughter face down in the water.

A neighbor dove in and pulled the little girl out. He immediately began giving her CPR before the paramedics arrived.

At the hospital, the child recovered over the next two days.

Even though she had probably been under water for almost four minutes, the little girl survived. They were fortunate that the mother's intuition and the neighbor's CPR training saved the little girl.

Some children have survived even after being under cold water for up to 30 minutes.

What occurs in drowning

Drowning typically occurs when the person gets fluid in the lungs. However, some drown not from getting water in their lungs but from spasms after they take the first gulp of water. This is called dry drowning and is actually suffocation.

Why people drown

Although some who drown don't know how to swim, many excellent swimmers drown each year. Simple fatigue is one of the most common factors in the drowning death of a good swimmer.

Use of alcohol or drugs impairs the swimmer and is a factor in 25 percent of drownings.

Inexperienced swimmers sometimes intentionally hyperventilate before diving so that they can remain under water longer. This removes carbon dioxide from their lungs. Then, during underwater swimming, they use up all their oxygen. Because the carbon dioxide levels are still low from the hyperventilation, there is no feeling of urgency to surface for a breath. Some pass out under water and drown.

Sudden illness like a seizure or a heart attack while in the water also contributes to deaths.

Injury to the head from a dive or from surfing or water skiing accidents are some of the other causes of drownings.

Use of alcohol or drugs impairs the swimmer and is a factor in 25 percent of drownings.

How to rescue

It is not wise to jump in to rescue unless you have been trained to do so.

If a pole, paddle, or flotation device is available, hold one end and extend it to the victim.

If the victim is not conscious, someone must go in to rescue him or her.

What to do when you get the victim out of the water

Most victims will regain consciousness when rescued. Vomiting and breathing difficulties are common.

If the victim has no pulse and is not breathing, begin CPR. This can be successful even if the victim has been in the water for some time. The human body is amazingly resilient, especially in cold water drownings below 70°F.

After exposure to cold water, watch for signs of hypothermia.

All victims of near-drownings should receive medical assistance since some will develop breathing difficulties or pneumonia in a few hours.

What to expect at the hospital after a near drowning

Victims are admitted for observation for pneumonia. Heartbeat irregularities or lung fluid overload may also occur but are not apparent for up to 24 hours. Chest x-rays are done, oxygen content of the blood is monitored, and occasionally antibiotics are needed.

What are the dangers of an electric shock?

Alternating Current (AC) can cause muscle spasms and stop the heartbeat. In fact, three people die every day from electrical injury. The degree of injury from an electric shock depends on the current and the voltage.

> A seven year-old was using the hair dryer in the bathroom. She accidentally dropped it into the tub where her four year-old sister was playing with floating animals.
>
> The younger girl screamed and then went silent.
>
> The mother rushed in from the bedroom and jerked the cord from the electric outlet. She dialed 911 on her cordless phone, pulled the child from the water, and began mouth-to-mouth resuscitation.
>
> The paramedics arrived, connected the child to the cardiac monitor, and used the defibrillator to shock her heart back to normal rhythm. Fortunately, she responded and was taken to the hospital for observation.

Injuries from electric shock

Electric shock can cause a variety of injuries, such as stopping the heart, burns, intestinal perforation, or liver or gall bladder damage.

Emotional support

Electrical shock can produce disorientation and confusion. If the victim is unable to communicate what happened, treat them for shock by lying them down, keeping them warm, and elevating their legs.

Ways to Prevent Electric Shock

• Children often fail to understand the potential problems of electrical outlets. An unused extension cord may look like a rope. By prohibiting play with extension cords, you minimize the risks.

• Power lines sometimes fall, leaving roads impassable. If the lines have fallen across your car, sit tight. Wait for assistance.

• A wet plug is a dangerous plug. Dry it off before using.

• Before using an appliance, look it over to make sure the cord is intact.

• Ground Fault and Circuit Interrupter (GFCI) receptacles automatically cut off whenever electric current is short circuited. Most new homes have them installed in crucial areas such as bathrooms and kitchens. If your family is not protected by GFCI receptacles, you can get these at hardware stores.

Electric shock can cause a variety of injuries, such as stopping the heart, burns, intestinal perforation, or liver or gall bladder damage.

What to expect at the hospital

Irregular heartbeats must be monitored for two days. Kidney failure occurs because of muscle damage so the victim will need blood tests for at least two days if severe damage occurs.

The victim may need an operation to remove large amounts of burned flesh.

How can I lower my child's temperature?

Fever is one of the ways our bodies fight illness. Fever can benefit health by killing certain bacteria or viruses. But fever can be harmful by causing seizures, dehydration, or chest pain or by breaking down muscles. For those reasons, it is better to keep the fever down and treat illness with medications.

Late one night, a small, crying child awakened his parents with a fever of 106°F. When they got to his room, he was having a seizure, or "fever fit," and later complained of an earache.

The parents sponged him off with cool water and gave him acetaminophen (Tylenol) bringing the temperature down to 101°F. Later at the emergency clinic, the family physician gave the parents antibiotics for the ear infection.

The parent's immediate action to bring the temperature down may have prevented the child from having another seizure or perhaps from having serious brain damage that could result from prolonged high temperatures.

Fever is a sign of some underlying problem. Because hundreds of diseases cause fever, it is not an indicator of one specific problem.

Temperatures of 105°F or greater are dangerous since serious brain damage may follow. Illnesses responsible for such high temperatures include meningitis, viral infections, malaria, a stroke, and other fatal illnesses.

An elevated temperature may not be due to fever if it occurs after prolonged heat exposure such as spending time in a hot tub or by jogging.

Important for children and young adults:

Don't use aspirin to reduce fever because it may cause fatal Reye's syndrome.

Detecting dangerous temperatures

Temperature is but one way to determine whether an illness is serious. A rule of thumb is that the following temperatures are not, by themselves, considered dangerous. Higher temperatures may be dangerous.

Under 3 months: 100.2°F
3 to 6 months: 101°F
Children 6 months and older: 102°F
Children over 6 months often develop temperatures of 104°F or higher at the onset of mild infections. But sometimes severe infections don't show temperatures over 100°F.
Adults: 102°F

What to do for a fever

For fever of 102°F or higher, try giving acetaminophen (Tylenol). Drinking cold water or sucking on ice chips can help bring the temperature down. Avoid milk since it might cause vomiting.

Use cool sponge baths for temperatures over 103°F if other measures don't work.

When fever is present, avoid excessive exertion.

One cause for fever is placing more blankets on a person who is chilling instead of giving acetaminophen.

An elevated temperature may not be due to fever if it occurs after prolonged heat exposure such as spending time in a hot tub or by jogging.

When a fever requires immediate medical care

Danger signs include breathing difficulty, bulging soft spot on a baby's skull, dehydration, diarrhea, drowsiness, earache, listlessness, low or high blood pressure, painful urination, rash or purple or red dots under the skin, seizure, severe cough, shaking chills, shock, sore throat, stiff neck, and unusual skin color.

What to expect at the hospital

If the person exhibits any of these symptoms, seek medical help right away.

The cause for the fever will be the focus of hospital care. If a high fever hasn't been responsive to home remedies, they will attempt to control the fever.

What are the signs of flesh-eating infections?

Every year, 85 people develop flesh-eating strep that destroys skin and muscle. While uncommon, these infections often cause death quickly. Because they are uncommon, few physicians have experience with them. To complicate matters further, flesh-eating strep can look like other diseases during the first few hours.

A 39 year-old department store manager developed pain in his arm. He had been playing softball for exercise and thought it hurt because he was out of shape. He saw his family doctor and was told to put ice on the arm and take ibuprofen.

That didn't seem to help. The pain got worse. After a couple of days, he went to the emergency room. The diagnosis was muscle strain as well.

About the same time, his wife and two children had strep throat and were given antibiotics.

The pain increased dramatically. He developed a red arm where the pain was, fever, night sweats, and chills. Again, he went to the doctor.

By this time, the arm was red, swollen, hot, and tender. It was obviously infected. An infectious disease specialist suspected necrotizing fasciitis and had a surgeon brought in to operate.

Necrotizing fasciitis means that the bacteria had destroyed the muscles and was quickly spreading. To stop it, muscles had to be amputated. Cultures taken of the muscle showed group A strep, the same strep his family had. In him it caused a different disease, though.

Strep comes in several types. Group A strep causes the worst infections. Besides strep throat, it causes rheumatic fever, kidney disease, and necrotizing fasciitis, called flesh-eating strep.

Reasons why different infections occur depend on the bacteria and the person infected. Unfortunately, it can't be predicted who will get the serious forms.

Necrotizing fasciitis refers to bacteria moving from muscle to muscle destroying everything in its path. Group A strep is just one of several types of bacteria that kills muscles in this way.

How do these infections start?

Flesh-eating strep infections usually begin by the strep penetrating the skin through a previous injury. A recent operation, a knife or gunshot wound, or other injury allows it to invade the body.

In some cases, there is no skin break, but a seemingly minor injury, such as a pulled muscle, allows the infection to begin. Different kinds of problems, in different people, lead to flesh-eating infections.

How to spot a flesh-eating infection

Flesh-eating strep infections are tender at first. Then, sensation is lost in the areas of dead muscles. The muscles just beginning to be involved are extremely tender. The skin will swell, turn red, and most people will have fever and sweats.

Treatment must be started at once. The dead muscle must be removed and antibiotics given. Even when a doctor recognizes the problem, there may not be enough time to treat it since death occurs quickly.

Other group A strep infections requiring immediate medical care

Strep doesn't have to be flesh-eating to be dangerous. Reportedly, Jim Henson, creator of the Muppets, suddenly became ill and died in only three days from Group A strep.

Older folks commonly develop another form of strep called erysipelas (airy-sip-a-lus) and have red, hot, tender skin with the infection moving through the skin over a period of hours. This, too, is an emergency.

Often less severe, impetigo is an infection on top of the skin with honey-colored pus draining from sores. This is usually found in children. Kidney problems can follow.

Flesh-eating strep infections usually begin by the strep penetrating the skin through a previous injury.

What to expect at the hospital

Cultures will be taken to show the bacteria, and intravenous fluids and antibiotics will be started at once.

An operation to remove dead and infected flesh is usually done if the infection is extensive or doesn't respond to antibiotics.

How can I keep my family from getting food poisoning?

A high school teacher purchased two pies, one butterscotch and one apple, from the day-old shelf of a local bakery. He took them home and his family ate some, although he didn't eat any himself.

Three hours after eating a piece of the butterscotch pie, his wife and eight year-old daughter became ill with vomiting and diarrhea. The daughter had eaten only one bite of the butterscotch pie and none of the apple pie.

They had vomiting and diarrhea several times per hour during the first hours. Then the mother began to feel better but the daughter continued to have problems. By the next day, the daughter was dehydrated. Her father gave her a drink which replaced the body's minerals lost in diarrhea. She began to feel much better over the next six hours.

It took one week for mother and daughter to recuperate and resume normal activities. Cream pies and potato salads are typical foods to cause staph food poisoning.

Watch for signs of food poisoning

Symptoms of food poisoning include nausea, vomiting, fever, chills, cramps, or diarrhea.

Food that smells or tastes normal may be contaminated. On the other hand, a foul smell or taste is a sign of food to avoid. For that reason, it is imperative to know that preparation and storage of food has been properly handled.

Advice for travelers

In restaurants with questionable sanitation, eat only thoroughly cooked foods, and drink bottled drinks with no ice. Pass up uncooked salads or raw food unless you peel it yourself.

Ways to Prevent Food Poisoning

Avoid touching cooked foods with hands contaminated by poultry. Diarrhea from this source may last several days.

Don't let anyone who has a draining sore on the hand prepare food. Even cooking does not inactivate staph toxins.

Use hot, soapy water to clean utensils, tables, and counter tops and remove bacteria.

Clean surfaces used to prepare uncooked meats before any other food touches the counter tops.

Store cooked foods at temperatures below 40°F.

Keep pets away from human food.

Wash hands before and after using the restroom.

Wash hands with soap and water before eating.

Avoid touching cooked foods with hands contaminated by poultry.

Foods unlikely to cause food poisoning

Meat was commonly salt cured in an earlier era. Salt cured meat remained edible for months without causing illness because salt and acid slow or prevent bacterial growth. However, if salt and acid do not penetrate deep into such foods, bacteria may grow.

Don't trust your pet to show unsafe foods

A pet's digestive tract is different from humans. What an animal can tolerate could cause sickness in humans. Also, unless the pet vomits or has diarrhea, an illness is difficult to know about. The pup lounging in the corner could have abdominal cramps.

Staph causes food poisoning outbreaks

A manufacturing plant notified the health department that several people were ill with vomiting and diarrhea. They had eaten lunch an hour before, and 28 of 38 employees felt deathly ill.

There were only two restrooms at the plant, and the first two people who became ill occupied them. Each had vomiting and diarrhea that wouldn't stop. Despite knocks on the doors and pleas from fellow employees to vacate, they couldn't come out.

Without anywhere to go, the co-workers vomited and had diarrhea outside the doors to the restrooms. It was an awful scene.

Why did it happen? The day before, they had a party with turkey, dressing, and all the trimmings. Lots of food was left over, so they saved it to have another meal the next day. They knew to keep it cold, so they placed it in a stairwell assumed to be unheated.

However, unknown to them, the stairwell was heated to 60°F, which kept the leftovers warm, allowing bacteria to grow. The food poisoning was due to staphylococcus. Staph food poisoning typically occurs 30 minutes to six hours after eating, and vomiting and diarrhea are symptoms.

Most often staph food poisoning is due to food preparation by someone with an infected sore on the hand.

Salmonella food poisoning

Why some get salmonella food poisoning

Salmonella commonly comes from eggs or poultry. If any food touches cutting boards contaminated by raw meat, salmonella or campylobacter can cause food poisoning.

People most likely to get sick from salmonella are those who do not have stomach acid. Medications which stop the stomach from making acid are Tagamet, Pepcid, Axid, Zantac, Prevacid, Prilosec, or Losec. Taking any of these can increase the risk of becoming ill if exposed to salmonella.

Illness From Food or Water		
Symptoms	**Disease**	**Source**
Fever, chills, abdomical discomfort, jaundice, dark urine	Hepatitis A	Human only
Fever, headache, gastrointestinal discomfort, vomiting, diarrhea	Viral gastroenteritis	Humans only
Fever, abdominal pain, diarrhea	Campylobacteriosis	Birds, cattle, cats, dogs, and humans
Watery diarrhea, vomiting, occasional muscle cramps	Cholera	Shellfish grown in brachish coastal waters
Fever, headache, constipation, appetite loss, nausea, diarrhea, vomiting, appearance of a rash	Typhoid fever	Humans only
Abdominal pain, fatigue, diarrhea (may be bloody), flatulence, weight loss	Amebiasis	Present in soil or vegetation due to fecal contamination
Diarrhea, abdominal discomfort	Cryptosporidiosis	Cattle and humans
Diarrhea, abdominal discomfort	Giardiasis	Water contaminated by animal or human excrement

Symptoms of salmonellosis

Diarrhea from salmonella begins 12 to 72 hours after eating contaminated food. Severity ranges from a few loose bowel movements to watery diarrhea every 10 to 15 minutes. Abdominal cramps, vomiting, fever, and chills sometimes occur with bloody diarrhea. Eventually, dehydration may cause the victim to collapse.

What to do

Keep the person hydrated with lots of liquid. Encourage drinking water or bouillon even if the victim doesn't want to. Commercial oral rehydration drinks, such as Pedialyte or Lytrea, for persons with *severe* diarrhea are available at the drug store.

Seek medical attention if dehydration occurs. Symptoms to watch for are light-headedness, not urinating or urinating very concentrated urine, high fever, and shaking chills.

Long-term danger from salmonella

Salmonella may spread to the bloodstream and infect the liver, kidneys, gallbladder, bones, or joints. People with sickle cell disease are at risk of developing bone infections.

Botulism food poisoning

A 33 year-old man had eaten home-style boiled eggs from a glass jug at a local mom and pop restaurant that featured these as a delicacy.

After eating the eggs, he became ill. He had friends take him to the hospital when he started having double vision. He couldn't focus his eyes or swallow. Fortunately, since he arrived for medical care early and received the botulism antitoxin, he survived.

Although the eggs were pickled in brine (salt water), the concentration of salt was too low to prevent bacteria from growing.

He was one of three people to develop botulism before the restaurant discarded the jug.

Why people get botulism

Botulism occurs most often in poorly canned foods. Harmful spores grow when food is canned without sufficient temperature or pressure. Following directions on pressure cookers is important when canning your own food.

A can that has a bulge suggests bacterial growth. Discard it without opening. The toxin and spores could contaminate your kitchen.

Traveler's Diarrhea

Common reasons for traveler's diarrhea

A 37 year-old telephone executive complained of cramping and diarrhea after returning from a trip to Mexico. She had stayed in a nice hotel, eaten at the hotel restaurant, avoided eating from street vendors, and used bottled water for drinking. She did use ice in her drinks, however.

She also swam in the hotel pool but didn't think the water looked clean. Additionally, she had a habit of singing in the shower.

Tap water in developing countries is often contaminated with E. coli causing diarrhea germs. With antibiotics, her diarrhea lasted only one day instead of seven.

Like many travelers, she probably had become exposed to contaminated water in four common ways.
• Brushing her teeth
• Singing in the shower
• Using contaminated ice
• Swimming in a non-chlorinated pool

What to do for food poisoning

Under 30 minutes.
Vomiting that begins within 30 minutes of eating or drinking is typically due to contamination with either metal or toxin. Induce vomiting if the person has not already vomited. Do not induce vomiting if the person has drunk an oily liquid or milk.

From 30 minutes to 6 hours
Symptoms of vomiting and diarrhea starting 30 minutes to 6 hours after eating are most often due to toxins from *Staphylococcus aureus*. Occasionally, symptoms begin a little longer than 6 hours later. Give fluids to prevent dehydration.

Between 12 and 72 hours

Diarrhea starting more than 12 hours after eating contaminated food is commonly due to salmonella, or campylobacter, often from chicken or turkey. Shigellosis comes from humans who fail to wash hands after using the toilet. Your health care professional will usually not prescribe antibiotics for salmonella and shigella. However, antibiotics are usually given for campylobacter.

Between 12 and 48 hours

Traveler's diarrhea is caused by *E. coli*. Diarrhea follows ingesting water by drinking, brushing teeth, or showering. Your health care professional can prescribe antibiotics as you prepare for travel. These stop the diarrhea in about one day, while not taking antibiotics allows diarrhea to continue seven days.

Between 12 and 36 hours

Botulism is rare and is the most lethal food poisoning. It comes from improperly canned food. The toxin of botulism is so potent that, in theory, two pounds could kill everyone in the world. Botulism begins with double vision, difficulty tracking with the eyes, numbness around the mouth, and problems swallowing. Seek medical assistance immediately. A shot of antitoxin may save the life of the victim.

Listeria is unique because it grows in the refrigerator. Milk, soft cheeses, and processed lunch meats are most often involved. It doesn't cause vomiting or diarrhea. Listeria produces meningitis and blood poisoning in babies, the elderly, cancer patients, and those with liver disease. Seek medical assistance for intravenous antibiotics.

Diarrhea from parasites begins one week to two months after eating contaminated foods. Parasites include ameba, cryptosporidium, or giardia. These cause persistent diarrhea for several weeks. Giardiasis causes gas with diarrhea. Seek medical attention. Oral metronidazole is often of benefit for ameba and giardia.

Is that arm broken?

Because a severe bruise and a broken bone may look similar, it is often hard to tell them apart. A bone may be completely broken, cracked in a hairline fracture, or chipped, yet maintain normal alignment.

The most severe fractures result in a deformed bone. If the bone breaks the skin, it may become infected, and heal slowly. Pressure on a nerve or blood vessel can cause additional damage.

An 18 year-old high school senior was scrimmaging with his football team. He was large but unusually agile. While he was carrying the ball, an opponent tackled him. He fell on his arm and heard a crack.

The pain was so severe he lay there and felt his arm swelling.

One of the coaches ran out with an ice pack and a splint while someone else called for an ambulance. They didn't move him since they weren't sure if he might have a neck or back injury.

The arm was splinted, and he had to wear a sling for the next several weeks. This took him out of the football games for the rest of the season.

How to recognize a fracture

Pain, bruising, and swelling are the most important indicators of fractures or sprains. Fractures are broken bones, while sprains mean the tendons or ligaments are pulled. At times, the difference is only found by x-ray.

Pain, bruising, and swelling are the most important indicators of fractures or sprains.

Yet some fractures show neither bruising nor swelling. Spine fractures cause pain without swelling or discoloration.

How to care for a fracture

Don't attempt to straighten disfigured bones. This could damage an artery or a nerve. Instead, place steady support on the injured area by making a splint using a board on one side of the injured area and wrapping it securely, but not too tightly. Leave the board until medically trained individuals can assess the injury.

How fractures occur

Trauma or falls are common causes of fractures. A fracture may result from minor injury when the underlying bone is weakened in osteoporosis, which happens in the elderly after menopause. Prolonged stress of walking or jogging for long periods when unaccustomed to doing so can cause a foot fracture.

What to expect at the hospital

Even before pain medications are given, the emergency physician checks for nerve or artery damage. Then the injured person receives pain medications and x-rays, and splints or a cast are put on.

What do I do for a heat illness?

It was July in Michigan. The temperature outside was a pleasant 74°F. An overweight 15 year-old desperately wanted to lose a few pounds so he could play football with the team in August.

He knew that exercising was a good way to lose weight, and he had heard that he might do it by sweating the pounds off. So, he turned up the thermostat to 85°F. Then in the basement, he worked out with weights.

His mother found him lying on the floor, dressed only in his shorts. He was sweating, felt weak and nauseated, and had a headache. The temperature was hot in the basement.

She immediately turned down the air conditioner, got some ice water from the refrigerator, and took his temperature. It was 102°F. He said that his muscles had been cramping, but he thought "no pain, no gain."

She had him begin sipping water, turned a fan on him, and stayed with him to provide reassurance. He had heat exhaustion. If she had not found him, he could have died from heat stroke.

How to care for heat cramps

Heat cramps, if ignored, lead to heat exhaustion. Heat cramps are painful spasms of the muscles due to loss of salt from the body.

Give the victim cool drinks and salty foods such as potato chips or pretzels.

Recognizing heat exhaustion

If not treated immediately, heat stroke follows and could cause death.

Heat exhaustion occurs with prolonged heat exposure (for hours) which dehydrates and depletes minerals from the body. If not treated immediately, heat stroke follows and could cause death. Symptoms include dizziness, excessive sweating, headache, muscle cramps, nausea, and weakness.

How to care for heat exhaustion

Lay the victim down in a cool shaded area and elevate the feet seven to twelve inches.

Give cool water or sports drink. If sports drink is unavailable, dissolve one-fourth teaspoon of table salt in a quart of cool water to make a sports drink substitute.

If there are no signs of improvement, seek medical help right away.

Recognizing heat stroke

Heat stroke begins when sweating stops and the skin feels hot and dry. If ignored, headache, dizziness, fast pulse, nausea, vomiting, or confusion may lead to collapse and unconsciousness. The victim's temperature is over 102°F. With prompt medical attention, 85 percent live. Seek assistance immediately.

How to care for heat stroke

Elevate the legs seven to twelve inches while sponging the victim with cool water. When the person regains consciousness, give cool water and sports drink.

What to expect at the hospital

Patients with heat stroke are admitted to watch for complications which include heart attack, liver or kidney failure, muscle damage, or coma.

Oxygen, intravenous fluids, and prompt reduction of body temperature are needed. For severe shivering, the victim may need intravenous medications.

Can I protect my family from spinal meningitis?

Meningitis is caused by many types of germs. The most feared type of meningitis is due to the deadly bacteria meningococcus. This can be transmitted from person to person so it creates panic in the community.

It can be prevented with immunization. However, few people have received the shot.

A 22 year-old university student phoned her mother saying she felt nauseated and was vomiting. She was going to skip classes the rest of the day.

The next morning, the mother tried to call her daughter. When no one answered, she convinced her husband that they needed to check on the daughter. The husband agreed to drive the three hours to the university.

Upon arriving, they found her apartment locked. Going around to a side window, the father saw his daughter lying unconscious on the floor.

Inside, they found she had a red rash all over her body, even on the palms of the hands. Her neck was stiff, and she felt hot with fever.

They rushed her to the local hospital. Meningococcal meningitis would have killed her within hours if the parents had not checked on her.

What is meningitis?

Meningitis is a severe infection in the blood stream and the lining of the brain caused by bacteria or viruses. The bacteria can exist in the body for a few days without harming the person, but once flu-like symptoms begin, it can cause death within 24 hours.

Recovery from viral meningitis does not require antibiotics, but recovery time is shortened if medication is taken.

The most common meningitis comes from viruses. There are three cases of viral meningitis for every case of bacterial meningitis. Recovery from viral meningitis does not require antibiotics, but recovery time is shortened if medication is taken.

On the other hand, meningococcal meningitis requires antibiotic treatment. Anyone exposed to this type of meningitis needs to take antibiotics to prevent getting meningitis as well.

Recognizing meningitis

Spinal meningitis symptoms include high fever, headache, vomiting, skin rash, rash on the palms and soles, and a stiff neck. A common complaint is, "This is the worst headache of my life."

Only rarely do rashes involve the palms and soles. Two emergencies caused by meningococcus and Rocky Mountain spotted fever both do this.

Avoiding meningitis

Those who eat, drink, or sleep with the victim are at risk. Droplets are passed by close contact such as sneezing, coughing, drinking from the same glass, or kissing someone who is infected. The person may not be sick at the time. Fully 95 percent of cases occur in people under age 25.

Can this type of meningitis be prevented?

A meningococcal vaccine is available but is not commonly used because of the low number of cases each year, but colleges have now begun to require its use.

What to expect at the hospital

The key is to get to the doctor as soon as the symptoms appear. Antibiotics must be given in the first few hours after onset.

After a quick but careful exam, a CT scan of the head may be needed. This is to be sure it is safe to do a lumbar puncture. The lumbar puncture removes fluid from the spine using a needle placed near the spinal cord. This allows a definite diagnosis for selecting the best antibiotics.

If there is a rash, the antibiotics will be started as a lifesaving measure even before the CT scan is taken.

Why does it hurt when I breathe?

There are two major types of pneumonia in adults—walking pneumonia and bacterial pneumonia. Walking pneumonia rarely requires hospital admission, while bacterial often does.

> A 35 year-old mother of two developed a cough and low grade fever of 100°F. Her two children had colds a week before, and all the kids at their day care had colds, also.
>
> The mother's cough was dry, meaning she didn't cough anything up. Her energy was reduced, and she didn't feel like getting out of bed. Her usual work as a paralegal was too strenuous.
>
> Her physician suggested taking erythromycin. However, he correctly told her that most people recover from walking pneumonia just as quickly without it. However, there may be less coughing later if an antibiotic is taken.

Typical symptoms for walking pneumonia are headache, cough without phlegm, fever, and fatigue.

The causes of walking pneumonia are viruses and virus-like germs. These are spread through families or day care centers.

Now contrast this with bacterial pneumonia.

A 40 year-old executive developed a shaking chill, temperature to 104°F, and a dry cough. He began to cough up phlegm a few hours later, and some had blood streaks. He felt horrible and was not able to get out of bed.

His wife rushed him to the emergency room later that evening where he was admitted to the ICU for severe bacterial pneumonia and treated with intravenous antibiotics. It was 10 days before he was able to go home and another 10 days before he could return to work.

Before modern medicine, bacterial pneumonia was known to cause a quick death in the elderly who might otherwise have had a slow, agonizing death. Sir William Osler, a famous physician, called it "the old man's friend." Oddly enough, Osler died from bacterial pneumonia just a few years after making the statement.

Symptoms of bacterial pneumonia

Typical complaints of bacterial pneumonia are fever, chills, being unable to get out of bed, coughing up phlegm that might be rust-colored or bloody, pleurisy (chest hurts with deep breathing), and shortness of breath.

Aspiration bacterial pneumonia

Another cause of pneumonia is sucking fluid or food into the windpipe. This occurs because someone has been unconscious due to drugs, alcohol, or disease. The name given to this type of pneumonia is aspiration pneumonia. This and bacterial pneumonia are usually more difficult to treat than walking pneumonia.

What to expect at the hospital

At the emergency room, an x-ray will evaluate the extent of pneumonia. Cultures show what bacteria or virus caused it, but the answer from these tests takes three to five days to complete.

Whether the pneumonia will be treated at the hospital or home depends on several factors. Hospital treatment occurs if the person is over the age of 70 or has a number of other factors which can increase the risk of dying.

Antibiotics used depend on the kind of pneumonia and the antibiotics currently effective. Today, many bacteria have become resistant to antibiotics. So newer, more expensive antibiotics are sometimes, but not always, needed. A few of the older ones like erythromycin, doxycycline, amoxicillin, and Bactrim may still be useful.

What was that stuff that made me sick?

Most poisonings occur in children between the ages of one and five. Boys are affected more than girls.

For adults, the most common reasons for unintentional poisonings are incorrectly identifying the contents of a container, having a mislabeled container, or failure to read or understand labels.

It was mid-July and 20 factory workers ate a lunch of tasty pork roast, boiled rice, cabbage, homemade biscuits, and soft drinks.

Within 30 minutes, five had abdominal cramps and nausea. During the next three hours, 12 others became ill with diarrhea, dizziness, and sweating. Their muscles started twitching, and nearly half had blurred vision. They were examined at the local hospital, and two were admitted.

In trying to identify the source of their illness, they found that only those who ate cabbage got sick.

The chef seasoned the cabbage from a can mislabeled "black pepper." He had not used it before this particular lunch.

Analysis of the black pepper found alicarb, one of the most potent pesticides in the United States. It is rapidly absorbed through the skin and is typically used as rat poison.

Common poisons and what to do about them

Of the 35 common types of poisons, the five most common ones are acetaminophen, household and garage products, iron, antifreeze, and aspirin.

How to care for a poisoning

The first step is to immediately call poison control.

The two types of poison victims are those who should not be made to vomit and those who should vomit.

Should not vomit

If the person is unconscious or has swallowed oil based poisons (such as oils, gasoline, or kerosene), don't make them vomit. They could get fluid into the windpipe, causing pneumonia.

If the person has swallowed a corrosive (like toilet bowl cleaner, detergent, or bleach) don't make them vomit. These burn on the way down and on the way back up. Dilute the poison by having the person drink plenty of water or milk.

If you don't know what they took, don't induce vomiting. It could be one of the above.

Should vomit

Induce vomiting if the person is conscious and you know they did not take one of the substances mentioned above.

Vomiting will usually not help if the poison was swallowed longer than three hours before.

Induce vomiting by placing the person's own finger in their throat or by using syrup of ipecac, available at the pharmacy. Follow directions on the label. Do not let the vomit choke them.

Why call poison control?

Use of charcoal helps to prevent absorption of many medications but not corrosive acids. Forcing fluids is great for some poisons, but harmful for others. Poison control centers have lists of drugs, antidotes, and which should be treated with fluids, milk, or charcoal.

What the physician will do for overdoses and poisons

Acetaminophen (Tylenol)
Untreated overdoses cause fatal damage to the liver. Immediate use of an antidote (acetylcysteine) saves the liver from severe damage.

Aspirin
Overdoses cause acid build up and very rapid breathing. Empty the stomach (up to 12 hours after swallowing). Charcoal may be used.

Antifreeze
Windshield washer solvent (methyl alcohol) causes blindness by damaging the optic nerve. Empty the stomach (up to four hours afterwards). Intravenous alcohol may be needed to give some protection.

Radiator antifreeze (ethylene glycol)
Radiator antifreeze crystallizes in the kidneys causing them to fail. Empty the stomach (up to four hours later). Intravenous fluids and intravenous alcohol may be needed.

Of the 35 common types of poisons, the five most common ones are acetaminophen, household and garage products, iron, antifreeze, and aspirin.

Iron
Iron tablet overdose causes bleeding of the bowels and brain, liver, and kidney damage. Pumping the stomach, even up to 12 hours later, may be necessary.

Mercury
Mercury causes tremor, loss of memory, and blindness. Chelation helps in some cases.

Lawn treatment additives
Insecticides cause muscle twitching, sweating, vomiting, and seizures. Atropine or praladoxime may help.

Herbicides

Herbicides cause bleeding and kidney failure. Special medications help.

Bleach

This causes swelling of the voice box, hoarseness (sometimes permanently), and damage to the esophagus. The stomach should be pumped by placing a tube into the stomach, not by allowing vomiting. Special medications help.

I think it's a seizure. What do I do?

Seizures are electric discharges in the brain that involve part or all of the brain. Some seizures affect only an arm or a leg. Others cause the entire body to contract.

A middle-aged man collapsed while grocery shopping. A nearby clerk rushed to call 911.

The man had a violent spasm. His arms and legs jerked uncontrollably as he began to froth at the mouth. After 30 seconds, his shaking subsided, but his eyes did not open.

Reacting quickly, the clerk checked for a pulse. Upon finding one, he turned the man's head to the side to prevent vomit from choking him.

The paramedics arrived shortly to take him to the hospital, and the man survived.

The stages of a grand mal seizure

People who have seizures are typically aware if they are about to have one. They have a premonition followed shortly by a moan or cry as the seizure starts. They fall, and their muscles contract. Then they stiffen, jerk, and lose control of bowel and bladder functions. Some bite or swallow their tongue.

How to help someone during and after a seizure

Have them lie down, if possible, before the seizure starts. Clear the area of harmful objects.

Before the seizure starts, place a rolled washcloth or handkerchief between the teeth to protect the tongue.

After the seizure, turn the person to the side to prevent getting vomit in the lungs. Allow sleep to follow.

Seek medical assistance if this is a first seizure, a seizure after a long seizure-free interval, or is different from usual seizures.

Be sure the person is taking seizure medications as prescribed and has not started a new medication that might interfere. This may require checking with their doctor or pharmacist.

People who have seizures are typically aware if they are about to have one.

What not to do during a seizure

Don't hold down the person down.
Don't try to keep the person from jerking.
Don't try to give CPR.

He hurt his head. How should I help?

Auto accidents are the most common cause of severe head injuries. Alcohol often plays a part. Most head injuries don't cause skull fractures but may injure the brain. If the skull is fractured, bleeding into the brain is more likely.

A 19 year-old was driving his pickup truck over a lonely road. Wanting to see how fast he could corner the next turn, he down-shifted, and sped into the turn. Unfortunately, the truck rolled, and the young man hit his head.

He was knocked unconscious by the impact. Fortunately for him, a vehicle was approaching from the opposite direction, and the driver was able to call for help on her cell phone.

Early effects of a head injury

Bruising, swelling, and bleeding in the brain are common after a head injury and can cause unconsciousness. Depending on the extent of these effects, permanent brain damage can result and make a young person look as though they've had a stroke.

If a skull fracture did occur, the victim could develop meningitis later. This would not be the contagious type of meningitis.

How to care for a victim of head injury

If you are first on the scene, be sure the victim is able to breathe and is not lying face down in water or on an object that prevents breathing. Don't allow the head and neck to be moved, but stabilize them to prevent the victim from being paralyzed in case there was a neck or back injury. Only qualified paramedics should change the position of the head and neck unless the victim would drown or suffocate otherwise.

If a skull fracture did occur, the victim could develop meningitis later.

Shock may occur, so getting immediate medical assistance is mandatory.

Why head injuries are serious

Common disabilities after head injury include inability to use arms and legs, to speak, or to see. Also, head injuries cause the brain to shrink, and sometimes epilepsy follows.

What to expect at the hospital

Before stitching up a laceration, skull x-rays are taken to look for a fracture. A neurologic examination along with CT scans and other tests assesses brain damage.

Even if the injured person is sent home, family members should help watch the eyes to be sure the right and left pupils stay equal in size. An early sign of problems is one pupil getting larger than the other. This requires instant medical attention to prevent death or permanent brain damage.

To relieve pressure on the brain, the person needs special medications or perhaps an operation to drain blood.

How can I keep from getting pregnant or getting AIDS?

A 19 year-old college student accepted a date with an older guy in one of her classes. On the first date, he was a gentleman. On the second date, he acted like a different person. He was mean and forced her to have sex. She tried to talk him out of it and pushed him away until he overpowered her.

Immediately afterwards, he left and she went to a friend's apartment. They took her to the ER.

Because this was termed "date rape," the personnel agreed to do the medical tests, but the investigating officer told her prosecution would be difficult.

Early effects of sexual assault

Psychic trauma. Psychic trauma is of utmost concern. After date rape, trust in persons of the opposite sex is tenuous. Fear of repeating the event is strong. After an anonymous attack by a stranger, getting into strange situations is emotionally draining.

Physical injuries. Sexual assault is usually more about injury and domination by the perpetrator than it is about sex. The victim may be harmed in a variety of ways, both externally and internally.

Late effects of sexual assault

Pregnancy. Women are rightly concerned about the possibility of pregnancy following vaginal penetration.

Sexually transmitted diseases. Any of the sexually transmitted diseases could follow such an assault.

Disease prevention

1. Pregnancy.

If the attacker cannot be dissuaded, sometimes he can be convinced to wear a condom. If not, and if there has been vaginal penetration, taking a high dose estrogen pill can prevent pregnancy. The ER can supply the pill, which the victim should take within 24 hours. An option for someone who takes oral contraceptives would be to take two days extra doses. Check with your personal physician.

2. Sexually Transmitted Diseases.

a. AIDS/HIV. If the attack was by someone HIV positive, acquisition of HIV can be greatly reduced by taking the following medications for one month: Combivir (zidovudine and lamivudine), one tablet twice daily, and Crixivan (indinavir), two tablets every eight hours. This reduces the chance of getting HIV by at least 80 percent.

b. Chlamydia. Chlamydia causes vaginal discharge and pelvic inflammatory disease in women and urethral discharge in men. Using doxycycline twice daily for one week provides effective treatment.

c. Gonorrhea. This also causes problems like chlamydia, but often the symptoms are much more severe. Patients can be treated with one 400 mg tablet of Suprax.

d. Syphilis. The VDRL blood test becomes positive if a person has been infected. A person may have symptoms or remain symptom free. When treated early, immediately after assault, a single injection of benzathine penicillin can cure or prevent syphilis.

e. Venereal warts. Some strains of the wart virus (HPV) don't cause warts but can cause cervical or penile cancer. The physical examination can catch it early, and treatment is effective.

> An option for someone who takes oral contraceptives would be to take two days extra doses. Check with your personal physician.

f. Hepatitis B. If a person has had the three dose vaccine, then protection is good. Otherwise, using the hepatitis B gamma globulin and vaccination can be helpful.

g. Others. There are more than 25 diseases that can be spread sexually. If symptoms develop later, return for a repeat evaluation.

What to expect in the emergency room visit

The physician will do a complete general exam including a vaginal exam to show presence of semen and sperm. If any identifying marks were made or if body hairs were left, this will be collected. Such evidence is used to prosecute the perpetrator.

Can anyone help me? I've been bitten.

In the United States, two main kinds of snakes are poisonous: coral snakes and pit vipers (rattlesnakes, copperheads, and cottonmouths). Fortunately, only 20 percent of people bitten by a poisonous snake are actually exposed to the snake venom.

On a scout trip, the troop was fishing along the rocky bank of a stream. A 15 year-old scout was not watching where he was walking. All at once, he heard a buzzing and felt a sting on his leg.

Looking down, the scout saw a snake. He screamed, jumped back, and kicked at the snake.

His scoutmaster sprang to the rescue and put a tourniquet around the leg. Several of the other scouts helped carry the boy to the van to transport him to the first aid station.

After a snake bite, capture and kill the snake to identify what type it is.

Rattlesnakes, copperheads, and cottonmouths all have slit-like eyes with poison sacs behind them. They also have long fangs.

The coral snake has rounded eyes but has poison sacs like other poisonous snakes.

Coral snakes also have black and red bands around the body, separated by yellow bands.

Remember this rhyme to recognize the difference between a poisonous coral snake and a non-poisonous king snake.

"Red and yellow, flee the fellow;
Red and black, venom lack."

Bites from the coral snake, the Mojave green rattlesnake, and the cobra may not produce symptoms until six hours later.

Symptoms may include blurred vision, problems with swallowing, eye lids drooping, increased salivation, and slowed breathing.

Bites from pit vipers cause swelling and muscle breakdown.

Up to 30 percent of bite victims who receive antivenom develop a serious fever, rash, and joint pain two weeks later.

What to do after a snake bite

Check the bite victim's pulse, blood pressure, and breathing.

Make sure bleeding is controlled.

Remove objects, such as rings and bracelets, which may be difficult to remove later after swelling occurs.

Keep the bite area below the level of the victim's heart. Immobilize as if it were broken.

Clean the bite with running water, soap, and a clean brush.

Cover with a clean cloth, and wrap with elastic bandage. Don't cut off circulation.

A commercial venom extractor can remove 25 percent of the venom in five minutes.

What to avoid after a snake bite

Never cut into a snake bite.

Never apply a tourniquet or apply suction.

(Authorities differ on the use of a tourniquet. The important thing is to avoid cutting off circulation if a tourniquet is used and to have a physician remove it. If you cannot get to a physician, do not use a tourniquet.)

Never put a cold or hot compress on a snake bite.

Never raise the bitten body part above the victim's heart.

Never give alcohol, aspirin, or pain medication.

Never delay medical care. Antivenom is most effective when given soon after a bite.

What to expect at the hospital

Antivenom, made from horse serum, reduces the damage done by the snake bite venom. However, up to 30 percent of bite victims who receive antivenom develop a serious fever, rash, and joint pain two weeks later. This is called serum sickness.

The dose of antivenom given depends on the symptoms. If there is pain and swelling, the victim will need small doses. Larger doses are needed for victims with nausea and numbness. Even larger doses are required when severe swelling, pain, bruising, twitching muscles, or a drop in blood pressure occur.

How should I care for a scorpion sting?

Scorpions are one to three inches long, yellowish, and mostly found in Texas, New Mexico, and Arizona along the Colorado River. Most scorpion stings are harmless, producing a small local reaction. However, some cause severe toxicity creating neurologic problems.

How to identify the sting of a poisonous scorpion

Light pressure on the site hurts intensely. This local tenderness lasts several days.

For more severe reactions, within 60 minutes of the sting, the victim becomes restless, jerks, sweats, has double vision, loses urine, is confused, salivates excessively, may have a seizure, and may wheeze or have difficulty breathing.

How to treat a scorpion sting

Apply ice packs to relieve the pain. (Don't place ice in direct contact with skin.)

Avoid getting the skin too cold.

Immobilize the affected area.

Do not apply a tourniquet.

My husband's having a stroke. How do I help him?

Stroke is the third most common cause of death, affecting one in 200 people every year. It occurs most often in men over the age of 60.

A 65 year-old man had just fixed two waffles for his wife and himself. After putting strawberries and maple syrup on them, he felt the onset of a headache.

He suddenly found himself on the kitchen floor, unable to move his left arm or leg. He noticed he couldn't speak clearly and just mumbled as he tried to call his wife.

His wife came around the corner and saw him. Noticing something was wrong, she asked, "Are you okay?"

He responded, "Yes, just help me to bed."

Instead, she said, "I'm going to call 911."

He tried to stop her because he felt that wasn't needed. The problem wasn't very serious.

Despite his insisting, she went ahead and called for help.

The ambulance got him to the hospital in a few minutes. A stroke was in process, and he was given a clot buster. Within hours, he was much better. Today he is completely normal.

Only because of the quick work of his wife and the emergency department staff can this man walk and talk today.

Steps to take if you suspect a stroke

Recognize the signs

A stroke occurs when a blood vessel in the brain bursts or blood flow is obstructed by a clot. Immediately, the brain swells and the lack of oxygen causes the nerves to malfunction.

The signs of a stroke vary depending on the location of the clot. Common signs include dizziness, intense headache, and weakness in the face, arm, or leg on one side of the body. It can also include mumbled speech, inability to see clearly, or loss of consciousness.

> Common signs include dizziness, intense headache, and weakness in the face, arm, or leg on one side of the body.

Call for help immediately

Much can be done for strokes, but immediate medical attention is crucial. Clot busters are highly effective in reversing the damage if used during the first three hours after the beginning of a stroke. So get help fast.

What to expect at the hospital

If clot busters are given within three hours after the beginning of a stroke, brain damage is often reversed. However, the clot buster is not without risks. These may cause unwanted bleeding or, rarely, even cause a worse stroke that would be fatal to the victim.

What is causing this rash and fever?

Three of the serious diseases from ticks are Lyme disease, Rocky Mountain spotted fever, and tularemia.

Each of these is named for a part of the country where it was discovered—Old Lyme, Connecticut; the Rocky Mountains; and Tulare County, California.

These diseases begin with fever and usually a rash.

Lyme Disease

A mother called her physician because she was concerned about her nine year-old son. He was suffering from symptoms similar to arthritis. Several children in her son's class were experiencing the same thing, and she found this unusual and troublesome.

Each of these children had a rash at the site where a tick had been removed. They developed more rashes, bull's-eye in appearance and about the size of quarters, scattered all over the body.

The children were treated with intravenous antibiotics while blood tests were run. The tests took 10 days to confirm Lyme.

Lyme is the most common disease from ticks in the country. This disease usually occurs between May and August in New England, the Midwest, and California.

What to expect at the hospital

A blood test will be drawn to see if antibodies are being made against Lyme bacteria. If they are, a Western blot test is done to be sure that they are specific for Lyme and not caused by some other infection.

The sick person will receive oral antibiotics such as amoxicillin, doxycycline, or intravenous Rocephin.

Problems typically requiring attention include skin rash, joint pains, nerve weakness, meningitis, or heart block.

Rocky Mountain Spotted Fever

A 14 year-old delirious boy was seen at the hospital with fever of 104°F, skin rash, and severe headache. His mother said he had not had any tick bites but had been picking ticks off his dog every night.

Match-head sized red spots were present on the palms of his hands and soles of his feet, two areas typical for Rocky Mountain spotted fever. The rash didn't itch and wasn't painful.

They admitted the boy to the hospital and treated him with the antibiotic doxycycline. By the next day he was better. After a week, he was able to go home.

Rocky Mountain spotted fever starts one week after the tick bite with light hurting the eyes, headache, fever, chills, muscle aches, and vomiting.

Rocky Mountain spotted fever starts one week after the tick bite with light hurting the eyes, headache, fever, chills, muscle aches, and vomiting.

The rash helps determine the diagnosis

Interestingly, Rocky Mountain spotted fever is not typically found in the Rocky Mountains today.

This disease is passed down from one generation of ticks to another. So if it is found in an area, it can be expected there again in the future.

Rocky Mountain spotted fever has been found nearly everywhere in the country, but the middle Atlantic states tend to have more than other areas.

This may be a fatal illness so it requires immediate attention. Patients go into shock without treatment.

What to expect at the hospital

Because Rocky Mountain spotted fever can progress rapidly, antibiotics must begin even before blood tests are back. Waiting could result in death. To make matters difficult, a person must be sick for a week before the blood test can become positive.

Tularemia

This disease is often called rabbit fever since rabbit hunters get it by nicking the skin when handling rabbits. It can also result from tick bites or from eating contaminated meat.

> A 39 year-old farmer went hunting with his 15 year-old son. They shot and skinned seven rabbits, placing the carcasses in the freezer to eat later.
>
> The farmer got a black spot on his thumb, and then developed fever. At the time he was examined, there were swollen glands just above his elbow and under the armpit on the same side of his body.
>
> He was started on the antibiotic doxycycline and improved after a few days.

Symptoms of Tularemia

Tularemia is found in the South Central states and occurs about three to five days after contact with a tick or rabbit. At the spot of contact with a rabbit, a sore appears and the glands get swollen and tender. If not treated promptly, about 10 percent of the victims will die.

What to expect at the hospital

The person will receive antibiotics at once while waiting for tests to check the diagnosis.

Why can't I keep anything down?

There are many causes of vomiting and diarrhea. Often a virus, or occasionally food poisoning, may cause these symptoms. Either vomiting or diarrhea may be a sign of a severe illness.

Generally, if only vomiting and diarrhea are present without pain or fever, use of home remedies for up to three days is prudent. But if there is a lot of either vomiting or diarrhea, dehydration may result. In these cases, medical assistance needs to help control the diarrhea or vomiting and find a cause.

A 23 year-old woman had been vomiting for two days. Despite drinking plenty of bouillon, tea, and Sprite, she wasn't getting any better. About 3 a.m. she vomited again. It looked like coffee grounds, and she felt light-headed. She had her brother rush her to the hospital.

At the hospital, a tube placed through her nose into her stomach flushed her stomach with ice water. Bright red blood was removed.

The coffee ground vomit showed she was bleeding in the stomach. Light-headedness is typical of either dehydration or hemorrhage.

What to do if someone is vomiting

If the person is unconscious and lying on their back, turn them to the side to keep them from choking. This is to prevent fluid from getting into the lungs, causing pneumonia.

When the person regains consciousness and stops vomiting, replace losses with water, bouillon, and sports drink.

What you can take for vomiting

Vomiting can sometimes be alleviated by using nonprescription medications such as meclizine. Sometimes eating dry crackers and apples can reduce vomiting.

Children should avoid milk for several hours or days and take clear liquids.

Children should avoid milk for several hours or days and take clear liquids.

Signs vomiting is serious

Sometimes vomiting indicates a serious problem. Seek immediate medical help for the following situations.

Vomiting along with abdominal pain or injury.

Vomiting after a head injury.

Vomiting is persistent or with fever.

Vomiting leads to dizziness, light-headedness, or fainting.

Vomiting with another illness. Vomiting with the flu or chicken pox can be an early sign of Reye's Syndrome.

Vomit is bright red with blood or shows dark material resembling coffee grounds.

Signs diarrhea may be serious

Diarrhea is black or bloody.

Diarrhea accompanies abdominal pain or fever.

Diarrhea persists or is very frequent.

Diarrhea leads to dizziness, light-headedness, fainting, or dehydration.

Diarrhea is due to food poisoning.

What you can take for diarrhea

Stop drinking caffeinated products, alcohol, laxatives, and milk products to let the bowels rest. Continue drinking other fluids.

Loperamide is available without a prescription. Follow the label.

Bacterial capsules (acidophilus with bulgaricus, thermophilus and bifidum) can stop many diarrheas by replacing bacteria in the colon.

I'm bleeding. Please get help!

Injuries to the chest or abdomen from gunshots, stabbings, or arrows are some of the most dramatic illustrations of emergencies.

A 47 year-old man was sawing firewood on a chilly autumn morning. He was in a hurry and was sitting on the limb he was cutting when his chain saw slipped. It ripped through his jeans and sliced his leg, causing a torrent of blood.

Instantly light-headed and nauseated, he made his way back to the truck and used his cell phone to call for help before he passed out.

He regained consciousness enough to realize he was losing blood, so he removed his belt and used it as a tourniquet, knotting it tightly around his leg above the injury.

He was rushed to the hospital where physicians found he had lost a lot of blood. They were able to repair the damage, but he'll always carry a long scar on his leg.

Injuries to the abdomen or the chest are more likely to cause death than those to the arms or legs, although these can cause serious bleeding or get infected.

What to do for a cut, stabbing, or nail injury

A knife or sharp object injures by separating tissues, allowing bacteria to enter the body. Clean the cut immediately with antibacterial soap and running water. This is not possible for deep stab wounds that close when the knife is removed. Yet if a dirty weapon was used, a physician may need to reopen the wound for cleaning. Seek medical assistance at once.

Stop the bleeding by placing pressure with a clean, dry cloth over the cut. Because of the risks of HIV, wear rubber gloves or plastic bags over the hands when working with someone else.

If direct pressure does not stop the bleeding, apply a tourniquet. Obviously, tourniquets aren't used for head, neck, chest, or abdominal injuries.

Any cut on the face requires special attention to limit scarring.

Caring for minor cuts at home

1. Wash with soap and water to reduce infections.

2. After washing, rinse again with water or hydrogen peroxide.

3. Do not apply iodine or merthiolate.

4. Apply Neosporin (triple antibiotic) ointment to reduce infections (unless allergic).

What to expect at the hospital

It is easier for the emergency physician to predict the damage done after a knife wound than a gunshot wound. Knife wounds can often be probed to determine the severity, thus avoiding operation.

Any knife wound to the chest below the nipples may have injured the abdomen as well as the chest, lungs, heart, or blood vessels. The victim may need extensive tests, including surgery.

If yellow fat can be seen, the cut is deep and requires sutures or steri-strips to close. Otherwise, infections are likely.

All wound victims will receive a tetanus toxoid shot if they haven't had the last shot within the past five to ten years.

After a dirty injury, if someone has not had tetanus shots, they must get two types of shots, tetanus toxoid and tetanus gamma globulin.

Why gunshot wounds are so destructive

Shotgun wounds are devastating at close range. When they are fired from nine feet away, 90 percent of victims die, even if they are rushed to the hospital.

A shotgun fired from 20 feet may cause pellets to penetrate the heart or liver.

A shotgun fired from 120 feet does not allow the pellets to penetrate far into the tissues. Obviously if an eye were hit, damage would be great. But if the belly wall was hit, serious damage is not likely for adults unless a large caliber slug was used.

The severity of a rifle or handgun wound depends on the size and speed of the bullet, where it hits, what it destroys, and whether the bullet stops in the body.

A handgun bullet with less speed does less damage than a rifle. A bullet with a soft-point or hollow-nose spreads out and causes much more damage to the victim.

What to do for gunshot wounds

Since gunshots cause internal injuries, seek medical assistance immediately. While waiting for medical assistance, there are a couple of things to remember.

If there is bleeding, control it by applying pressure directly over the wound with a clean cloth. If swelling begins, elevate the swollen area above the heart.

What to expect at the hospital

Visible particles will be removed from the wound.

The victim may need x-rays or CT scans to assess the damage.

Blood tests will show how much blood was lost and whether a transfusion is needed.

If the bullet entered the chest or abdomen, the victim might require an operation to search for tears that could bleed later or for an intestinal leak that could cause an infection.

How to know if the wound is infected

Even if contaminated with bacteria, wound infections will not be apparent for several hours or even up to a few days.

Shotgun wounds are devastating at close range. When they are fired from nine feet away, 90 percent of victims die, even if they are rushed to the hospital.

An infected wound may drain pus or be red. Other signs that the wound is infected include chills, fever, or red streaks. Red streaks up the arm or leg mean blood poisoning, which is dangerous.

An infected abdominal or chest wound lacks the red streaks but is usually even more life-threatening. Pain, fever, chills, or night sweats are typical.

To Order Additional Copies of This Book

To order additional copies of this book, complete the form below and fax or mail to 90MinuteBooks.

Fax to: 770-801-8865

Mail to: 90MinuteBooks
Book Orders Dept.
1365 Ashwood Court, Suite 300
Smyrna, GA 30080

Cost:

Quantity	Price	Shipping Per Book
1	$11.95	$3
5+	$10.95	$2
25+	$9.95	$1
100+	$6.50	$ .25

❑ Yes, I wouild like to order *When Seconds Count*. Please send me _____________ copies of the book.

Method of Payment: ❑ MC ❑ VISA ❑ AMEX
❑ COD (Please add $7)

Card Number _______________________________________

Expiration Date _______________________________________

Cardholder _______________________________________

Ship-to Address

Name _______________________________________

City _______________________________________

State _______________________________________

Zip _______________________________________

Phone _______________________________________

www.ingramcontent.com/pod-product-compliance
Lightning Source LLC
Chambersburg PA
CBHW031309060726
47590CB00003B/1122